HOMOEO...
FOR W...

(Bought with The gift
token given to me by M&S).

Rima Handley was born and educated in Blackpool then went to Oxford University where she studied medieval English language and literature. She taught medieval literature at the universities of London and Newcastle-upon-Tyne for several years and then gave up the academic life to train and practise first as a homoeopath and subsequently as a psychotherapist. She now combines the practice of both psychotherapy and homoeopathy. She was co-founder of the Northern College of Homeopathic Medicine, one of the first homeopathic training colleges to be established in the UK, and still takes an active part in the running of the College. She has written two other books about homoeopathy, *A Homeopathic Love Story*, a biography of the founder of homoeopathy, Samuel Hahnemann and his wife Melanie, the first woman homoeopath (published by North Atlantic Books in 1990), and the second, *In Search of the Later Hahnemann,* published by Beaconsfield Press. She now practises in Newcastle and Kendal.

HOMOEOPATHY FOR WOMEN

Rima Handley

M.A., D.PHIL., DIP.ADV.PSYCHOSYNTHESIS, F.S.HOM.

Thorsons
An Imprint of HarperCollinsPublishers

For Nan

Thorsons
An Imprint of HarperCollins*Publishers*
77–85 Fulham Palace Road,
Hammersmith, London W6 8JB

Published by Thorsons 1993
1 3 5 7 9 10 8 6 4 2

© Rima Handley 1993

Rima Handley asserts the moral right to
be identified as the author of this work

A catalogue record for this book
is available from the British Library.

ISBN 0 7225 2781 0

Typeset by Harper Phototypesetters Limited,
Northampton, England
Printed in Great Britain by
HarperCollinsManufacturing Glasgow

CONTENTS

Carmaris?

Acknowledgements

I am grateful to many people for reading this book during the time I was writing it and offering support and suggestions: Linda Anderson, Melissa Assilem, Naona Beecher-Moore, Amanda Bingley, Diana Clarke, Christine Conyers, Caroline Grist, Julia Haskell, Glynis Ingram, Vivienne Morris, Gabriela Rieberer, Beryl Sanderson. I am also very grateful to Connie Driver for doing so much to give me the time to write.

I have learnt most about how to write this book from my women patients, who have helped me without knowing it.

Rasta's support has been invaluable.

Note to the reader:
Properly used homoeopathic remedies are safe and without side-effects. If in doubt consult a qualified practitioner. Neither the publishers nor the author accept responsibility for any effects that may arise from giving or taking any remedy included in this book.

Preface

These days, health is a common theme in books, articles and television and radio programmes. Women in particular are keenly interested in the subject both for their own sake and that of their families. This book has been written especially with them in mind for it is they who bear most of the responsibility for the family's health. It is often women who are most exposed and vulnerable to the frustrations and inadequacies of orthodox medicine since they have more contact with it due to the high level of medical intervention in menstruation, childbirth and child rearing.

In the last fifty years or so the enormous advances made by orthodox medicine in the field of surgery and drugs have had some remarkable effects. Many conditions that were regarded as incurable have become tamed and many once fatal diseases are now almost non-existent. However, the development of powerful drugs has brought its own problems and there are probably as many people suffering from their side-effects as there are who have benefited from them. Women are becoming aware of such things. They feel increasingly powerless and want to regain some sense of self-sufficiency in matters of health, some ways of taking charge of their own health.

Homoeopathy is one of the safest and most effective forms of medicine that has ever been discovered. Everyone who turns to it is amazed and delighted at how well it can work and how simple the process of cure can seem. If you have ever experienced the relief of giving a colicky baby a single pill of *Chamomilla* and watching her change from an explosion of bad temper and distress into a quiet and happy little girl you will know what I am talking about, just as you will if you have ever taken *Arnica* after a fall, and been amazed at the speed of recovery: sometimes it seems like magic.

Interest in homoeopathy and other forms of alternative medicine has increased to an enormous extent over the last few years. More and more people are consulting homoeopaths and naturally would like to be better informed about the kind of medicine they are using. Homoeopathic medicines are available over the counter in health food stores and pharmacists and yet there is little information offered about how to use them.

Homoeopathy is a very safe form of medicine: it uses remedies made from animal, vegetable and mineral substances prepared in such a way that they are powerful without being toxic. If a child were to swallow a bottle full of tablets there would be no ill effects. Homoeopathy is highly effective in curing a wide range of illnesses, from minor health problems to serious conditions.

This book explains clearly the principles and philosophy of homoeopathy, so different from those of orthodox medicine, and gives a readable explanation of how homoeopathy was discovered, how it works, how modern homoeopaths prescribe and how you yourself can use it to improve your own and your family's health. It is designed to show you how to prescribe homoeopathic medicines successfully in simple cases, in some of the common illnesses and problems with which you may be faced from day to day as well as to give a fuller understanding of this kind of medicine so that you will be able to appreciate when it may be able to help you in more complex ways, even if you do not wish to prescribe yourself.

The book covers a wide range of conditions, from emotional

problems to conditions affecting the elderly, children's illnesses, and problems associated with menstruation, pregnancy and menopause. By the time you have read it and absorbed its information you should not only be a competent prescriber in first aid and simple conditions, but also have a real understanding of the holistic nature of homoeopathy, its important principles and many of its commonly used medicines. The material is centred on the use of a small number of easily available remedies which you can buy and keep in stock so as to be ready for all eventualities.

Once you have become interested in this fascinating subject you will find that there are self-help homoeopathy classes held in many parts of the country. Look for details of these in your local library and take an even deeper interest. There are also training colleges all over the country where you can take such interest further.

PART ONE

PART ONE

Chapter One

─────

LIKE CURES LIKE

Homoeopathic remedies are made from very tiny and highly diluted amounts of the substances after which they are named. It is safe to prescribe for yourself in the low strengths suggested in this book. If you prescribe for yourself and choose the wrong remedy it simply won't act; it won't have any other effects.

Homoeopathy has been around for over 200 years now. It was 1786 when its discoverer, the German doctor Samuel Hahnemann, first put into words the basic principle of the new medicine: *Similis similibus curentur*, which is usually translated as 'Like cures like' though it actually means something more like 'Let conditions be treated by things which are similar.' With this statement Hahnemann turned contemporary medicine on its head.

Whereas orthodox medicine tries to cure illness by treating it with substances intended to suppress the symptoms of the illness, to hide them, homoeopathy tries to cure illness by treating it with substances intended to increase the symptoms slightly, to bring them out more clearly, in order to galvanize the body's self-healing system into action. The idea was that under the pressure of a further disease, similar to the one it already had, the body would respond by throwing off both the original and the artificially added disease. This is why this form of medicine is called homoeopathy: the word is derived from the Greek *homoi-*, similar + *-pathos*, suffering.

Hahnemann's discovery was one of those amazingly simple reversals of the established truth which often take hundreds of years to be accepted. What he had noticed was that intermittent fever (malaria) was one of the very few diseases which could be cured by contemporary medicine. It was conventionally treated with the eighteenth-century wonder drug cinchona bark (from which quinine is derived), and Hahnemann began to wonder whether the reason for the success of the treatment was that cinchona bark was capable of causing very similar symptoms to those produced by malaria. To test his theory he took a few doses of the drug daily until he himself began to suffer from its poisoning effects, which, to his great delight, turned out to be similar to the symptoms of malaria.

This experiment confirmed the suspicions aroused in him a year earlier, when he had realized that mercury, the only drug that could make any headway against syphilis, itself produced very similar symptoms to those manifested by that terrible venereal disease which was rampant throughout Europe in the eighteenth and nineteenth centuries. In fact, because mercury was used in the treatment of a great many diseases in the eighteenth century, and because it caused symptoms similar to those of syphilis, it was frequently difficult to tell whether a patient was suffering from the disease or from poisoning by the mercury.

Hahnemann was thrilled and excited by his discovery. Once he had tested the cinchona bark on himself he began to draw in his friends, relatives and students to test many other drugs until he was satisfied that his theory could be generalized. In the first years after his breakthrough these helpers took repeated doses of (often poisonous) substances already used in contemporary medicine, substances such as aconite, arsenic, belladonna, mercury and silver nitrate. They did so in pursuit of Hahnemann's burning desire to establish the range of symptoms which each of these might cause and therefore cure.

These were the first 'provings', experiments in which a number of (more or less) healthy people took doses of drugs over a long enough period of time to elicit the symptoms in themselves. These 'provers' described their experiences in minute detail and such descriptions formed the basis of the 'drug picture' used to establish the range of symptoms capable of being caused by that drug, and hence the similarity of these to the symptoms existing in a sick person.

This is the first principle of homoeopathy. What a substance can cause it can also cure and if it cannot cause it, it cannot cure it. In practice then, if Hahnemann had a patient who was suffering from scarlet fever, he would not give a drug to bring down the fever, but might use a remedy called *Belladonna* which, in its crude form, has a tendency to cause a high fever with hot red skin and burning sensations. When given to the patient with fever, the body would feel further threatened and respond with an effort to overcome the fresh attack: in so doing it would activate its own self-healing powers and begin the process of getting well again.

This observation was only the beginning. Many years of experimentation and practice were to follow before Hahnemann was satisfied with his system: indeed he never was completely satisfied with it, and carried on experimenting until the very end of his life in 1843 when he was 89 years old. The experimentation and practice has gone on continuously since then in many parts of the world, and homoeopathy is now far more sophisticated and complex than it was in Hahnemann's day. However, it is still based on that one simple principle: cure is brought about by treating the person with a substance capable of causing symptoms similar to those she is showing when ill. Whatever the illness, the cure for it lies in finding the substance which is capable of producing effects as similar to the symptoms of the diseased person as possible, and in giving it to that person in order to activate the self-healing powers of the body. All cure comes from within the patient: it is not the medicines themselves which cure, they merely activate a healing reaction within the body.

The Body's Self-healing System

All natural medicines make use of the self-healing powers of the body. We know that we have a self-healing system: we know that if we are in reasonably good health cuts heal by themselves, colds come and go without much trouble, children recover from chicken pox with only rest and sleep. As long as we are healthy we can easily get over many of the complaints we contract, and we never even catch many of the things that are around. The surface of our bodies is covered with germs all the time, but most of these gain no power over us as long as we are fit. It is when we are not fit, when we are tired or stressed or weakened by a poor diet, that we start to catch everything and that it takes us longer to get over the illnesses.

Nowadays, in our culture we call the self-healing system the immune system or the immune and defence system. At different ages and in different places many other names have been applied to it. In India it is called *prana*, and identified with the breath of life, in Japan and China a similar concept is called *chi*: the balancing of *chi* energy is the basis of acupuncture and shiatsu. Both these concepts include a wider and deeper vision of the human organism than the Western concept of the immune system, but we are probably all talking about the same thing.

Hahnemann, along with his contemporaries, relied at first on the healing power of nature alone. Later, however, he came to realize that the power of nature was not enough by itself to cure disease, at least chronic disease, disease which is deeply embedded in the system and lasts a long time. Human reason needed to be introduced to awake and direct the dormant powers of the self-healing system, which he called the vital force, an energetic force inherent in the body, which both included and transcended the healing power of nature.

The body's self-healing system is maintained, first of all, by the traditional old-fashioned methods of eating healthy food, getting plenty of exercise and rest and living life as free from the pernicious effects of stress as possible. All this is easier said than done. Often we get caught in a vicious cycle, and this is where homoeopathy can help. Homoeopathy can step in and improve our general level of health, boost the self-healing powers of the system and thus enable us to take action about the diet, the exercise, the lifestyle. It can also do much more than lifestyle and diet in a number of cases.

Nowadays the self-healing powers of the body are coming under increasingly severe attack from a variety of pollutants. There are many 'new' illnesses which clearly strike directly at the immune system: M.E. (myalgic encephalomyelitis), *Candida* infestation and AIDS, for instance. In conditions such as rheumatoid arthritis or allergy (called auto-immune diseases) the self-healing system has even turned against its own body, so confused has it become.

All such diseases involve a severely weakened immune system which is simply unable to respond effectively to the invading illness. It is now more important than ever that we discover ways of boosting and balancing the immune system for ourselves, ways of taking back some control over our own health. It is looking very much as if it is some of the very achievements of orthodox science and medicine in the twentieth century that have contributed to the widely-evidenced breakdown in the immune systems of many people: antibiotics, drugs of other sorts and chemicals, both in food and in the air, have all been implicated.

Homoeopathy seeks to cooperate with and strengthen the immune system, and its main agent in this is the remedy whose symptoms most closely match the symptoms of the sick person, the *simillimum*, as it is called. Giving the *simillimum* supports the immune system, helps realign the self-healing powers of the body and strengthens our own capacity for maintaining health.

Chapter Two

———

THE MEDICINES

Hahnemann investigated nearly two hundred medicines before he died. Now, 150 years later, there are nearly 3000 medicines available for use by homoeopaths. They have been made from an enormous variety of sources including plants, trees, minerals, metals, disease substances and modern chemical drugs.

In the early days of homoeopathy most of the remedies were made from plants used in botanical medicine, plants such as aconite, belladonna, chamomilla, cinchona and pulsatilla; other substances in use in contemporary medicine were also pressed into service: arsenic, mercury, magnesium and nitric acid, for example. Hahnemann was a chemist as well as a doctor and he was therefore able to devise methods of making metals into medicines: gold, silver and platinum are all used in homoeopathy.

He was also quick to see the potential in substances which had not been used before then in medicine. Sepia, the brown inky disguise put out by fish of the squid family, was tried as a remedy after Hahnemann noticed that a severely depressed painter friend had the habit of sucking his sepia-covered brushes. Through speculating as to whether his friend's depression had been caused by this practice, Hahnemann came upon what was to become one of the most important homoeopathic remedies for people suffering from a whole range of symptoms associated with depression, including apathy, frustration, irritability and exhaustion.

Since Hahnemann's time, many other substances have been brought into use. Several exotic plants were introduced by the early American homoeopaths: Cimicifuga, Gelsemium, Ipecacuanha and Phytolacca, for instance. Remedies have also been made from charcoal, salt, bee stings, snake venom, oyster shell, nuts and modern drugs. In fact, anything at all can be used as a homoeopathic remedy as long as we know what symptoms it can cause and therefore cure. All the remedies in common use in modern times have been tested in the same kind of experiments as were originally devised by Hahnemann.

The evidence from these provings is supplemented by evidence from the literature about the poisoning effects of some of these substances, and by evidence from clinical practice. Many of the early homoeopaths took great personal risks to discover the symptoms of remedies. Constantine Hering, who explored the jungles of South America in search of likely remedies, paralysed his left arm for life while testing the venom of the Brazilian bushmaster snake, *Lachesis*.

Of course, this will not happen when taking remedies derived from these substances because they are taken in a very highly diluted form. It is impossible to be poisoned by a homoeopathic remedy.

We gain an enormous amount of information about each remedy from all these sources. We gain not only in amount, but in depth and scope of information from the fact that the reports are all based on the effects of the drugs on *people*: we therefore have access to knowledge about the subjective and psychological effects of the drugs. The provers noted such things as pains that felt like ants crawling on them, sensations as if they had a splinter in their throat, feelings of panic or despair, desire to laugh for no reason, pains in the joints that shot from one side of the body to the other, stomach pains which were better for eating indigestible food. They noted everything that happened to them while taking the drugs; their personal reports, their subjective accounts of their sensations and feelings while affected by the substances, form the core of the remedy picture. This is one of the reasons that homoeopathy is so exciting, because we can take advantage of all these hints and feelings and sensations which orthodox medicine has to ignore because it cannot use them.

The descriptions of all these remedies are collected in volumes referred to as *Materia Medica*. There are many varieties of these, ranging from Hahnemann's original head-to-toe detailed listing of every symptom produced by the provers to the more interpretative and psychologically informed pictures constructed by modern homoeopaths. A remedy picture is basically an attempt to give some form to the overpowering mass of detail provided by the provings and poisoning reports: it is an interpretation designed to bring understanding.

The *Materia Medica* in this book includes pictures of some thirty remedies. This might not seem a large selection from 3000, yet these thirty are probably the ones which are most widely used. Most of the remainder have a quite specialized application and are only used at all frequently by professional homoeopaths treating chronic illness. In my short descriptions I have concentrated on trying to communicate a general picture of each remedy, a picture which includes most of the symptoms characteristic of or special to each remedy.

If you try to absorb all the details of a remedy at once, you will sink without trace under a mass of detail. The provings of some of the major remedies have brought out thousands of symptoms in all areas of the body. Reading a complete picture of a remedy is like looking at one of Pieter Brueghel's paintings: there is far too much going on to be able to take everything in. Every time you go back to the picture you will find something else in it. However, the fact is that if you have any knowledge at all of what their paintings look like, you will never mistake a painting by Brueghel for one by Monet. You know straight away that Monet would not have painted a dark people-covered icy lake and that Brueghel would not have painted a light water lily-covered lake. Without being an art critic, you have unconsciously absorbed what is characteristic of the style of each painter. Likewise you will always be able to tell the difference between a blackbird and a robin, even if you know nothing about birds. You see what is characteristic about them, in this case colour and, to a lesser extent, size. It is the same with remedies.

If you look, for instance, at the picture of *Pulsatilla* in the *Materia Medica* you'll find that a person needing this remedy when ill is likely to be weepy, clingy and in need of company. She is also likely to be chilly, but at the same time uncomfortable in a stuffy room and quite badly affected by heat. She may faint easily. She won't apparently want anything to drink.

If you look at the picture of *Arsenicum* you will see that a person needing *Arsenicum* is also likely to feel better for company, but will not cry so easily; she will be meticulously tidy and precise in thoughts, attitudes and dress. She too will be a chilly person but she will feel better for being in a warm room or exposed to direct heat. She will be inclined to be thirsty, drinking little but often throughout the day.

A person needing *Natrum mur* will want to be on her own, will definitely not want sympathy from others and will certainly not let them see her cry. She won't have a marked temperature preference but will be quite thirsty. You might notice that her bottom lip is cracked in the middle.

A person needing *Lachesis* will probably be very intense and moody, very talkative and enthusiastic. She'll be easily affected by the heat and won't want anything tight round her neck or waist.

These sketches attempt to record the symptoms which are characteristic of each remedy, and most of which must be present in order for that remedy to be required. A picture of a single tree probably could not have been painted by Brueghel and a bird with a red breast cannot be a blackbird. *Pulsatilla* cannot be comfortable in a warm room and *Arsenicum* cannot be happy alone when ill.

Within the remedy pictures these characteristic symptoms are in fact the ones which most (in some cases all) of the provers experienced while taking the drug and they are also the symptoms which have been most frequently cured in clinical practice through the use of that remedy. So these symptoms are very definitely ones which can be caused and cured by the remedy. It is important to remember that many less strongly-emphasized symptoms have not been included and yet may be cured by the remedy. It is also important to remember that the remedy pictures included in this book are attempts to abstract sketches from vast oil paintings and that there is bound to be an element of subjectivity here: no two sketches of one oil painting will select and emphasize the same details.

Remedy pictures include a wide range of symptoms, some of which are clearly unhealthy: difficult breathing, pain in the right abdomen, heavy bleeding are some examples, while others seem to be scarcely more than character traits: bad-tempered in the morning, reserved or weepy, for instance. Homoeopaths form what is known as a *constitutional* picture of both patients and remedies. They consider that each person has a basic way of being in both health and disease which is best reflected in a single homoeopathic remedy picture. This way of being is referred to as the constitutional 'type' or picture.

So a *Pulsatilla* 'type' would be generally sociable, pleasant, easily emotional, chilly and thirstless whether she was ill or not, and these 'symptoms' would all be part of her picture. When ill she might develop catarrhal symptoms more readily than other 'types' might, and would tend to experience nausea after eating fatty food, have poor circulation, and trouble with her veins. A *Phosphorus* 'type' would be very sociable and entertaining, crave fish and chocolate and be a little on the chilly side. When ill she would be likely to develop symptoms in her chest or symptoms associated in some way with the loss of blood.

A person might conform to this remedy picture as a norm, her general way of being might correspond to it all the time in health, or she might fit a particular remedy picture only when suffering from an acute illness. That is to say that a person may be *generally* sensitive to and susceptible of being helped by a particular remedy, her constitutional remedy, or *temporarily* sensitive to it in her current style of illness. It is when the remedy matches both states that it acts most deeply. It is sometimes assumed that a person will display only one constitutional remedy picture throughout life; however, this is very rarely the case. Most people conform to the pictures of a number of closely related remedies at various times during their lives.

This book is concerned mainly with the treatment of acute and minor illnesses. Homoeopathy can also treat chronic illnesses, but these are best left to a homoeopath. Acute illnesses are those which come and go of their own accord if the immune system is strong enough. Children's illnesses like measles, mumps and chicken pox are acute illnesses in this sense, so are stings, burns, colds, flu and acute cystitis. Repeated attacks of any apparently acute or non-serious illnesses, including bad reactions to stings, imply an underlying chronic condition which could benefit from care by an expert homoeopath.

The purpose of this book is to make plain the principles of homoeopathy so that you can treat yourself in acute conditions and have an informed understanding of the treatment a professional homoeopath is likely to undertake in chronic conditions. Successful prescribing for acute and mild conditions can give you a sense of control and an appreciation of the possibilities of homoeopathy. You can then go on and get more experienced help for other conditions.

Chronic conditions are long-standing illnesses which cannot get better by themselves. These can vary in kind too: some are life-threatening in their acute episodes, such as colitis, others such as persistent catarrh, thrush, piles or dandruff are not so serious in themselves, but they do indicate the presence of a deeper disorder which needs to be addressed. Others are somewhere between the two: arthritis or psoriasis, for example, which are not immediately life-threatening but cause a great deal of distress.

Homoeopathy can be successfully and simply prescribed in the way outlined in this book because it relies so much on matching observable symptoms of both remedy and disease. But to prescribe successfully in chronic disease, a much greater understanding of the total disease process is needed.

You can discover the whereabouts of the trained homoeopaths in your area by writing to the Society of Homoeopaths for a list of registered homoeopaths or by contacting the homoeopathic training college nearest to you. The British Homoeopathic Association has a list of doctors who use homoeopathic medicines. See Appendices 2 and 3 for these addresses.

Chapter Three

FORMING A PICTURE
OF THE PATIENT

As we have seen, the successful prescribing of homoeopathic remedies relies on matching the picture of the remedy which will cure to the picture of the person who is ill. The picture does not have to match exactly, it just has to be similar; the more similar, the better the chance it has of exerting its catalytic effect on the patient's self-healing system. So the homoeopath's first task is to establish a picture of the patient: what are the symptoms?

A homoeopathic symptom picture clearly encompasses more aspects of the patient than those which orthodox medicine associates with disease. It attempts to depict everything of significance that is taking place within the patient at the time of the illness. Whatever is happening is an expression of just one state of dis-ease, one illness. All the symptoms present are related to each other, expressing a single mind-body condition. Everything about the patient is or may be a clue to the remedy.

Supposing your child has developed an earache. We know that she has pain in her ear. That symptom alone would lead us to a lot of remedies. *Aconite, Belladonna, Chamomilla, Hepar sulph, Merc sol, Pulsatilla, Silica* and *Sulphur* might all have pain in the ear. What else do we know? Is she crying or is she cross? Is she chilly or is she hot? Does she have a red face or a pale face? Is she hungry or has she gone off her food? Anything which is a change in her is important, and the more marked the change the more important it is as a symptom.

Let us imagine that your child has earache in which the area around the ear is hot and red; the child herself is also quite hot and red in the face and she is bad-tempered from the pain, which came on quite suddenly. The pain is improved when the ear is warmed. This child needs *Belladonna*, whose characteristic symptoms are sudden onset, redness, burning and bad temper. If she had had all the same physical symptoms but had been more restless, anxious and fearful rather than bad-tempered, and if the pain had got worse when the ear was warmed and the child herself was thirsty, you might have decided to give her *Aconite*. If she had not been quite so feverish and had been tearful and clingy, not wanting you to leave her, and if she had been uncomfortable from the warmth of the room, wanting a window open, then the remedy might have been *Pulsatilla*. Always look at the bigger picture, as whole a picture as possible.

If your child had been hot, very red in the face and bad-tempered suddenly and these symptoms did not accompany earache but, for example, a cold or measles, or one of those mysterious fevers of childhood, the remedy would probably still have been *Belladonna*. And if she had been tearful and clingy, not wanting you to leave her, uncomfortable in a warm room, then the remedy would probably have been *Pulsatilla*, whatever the particular physical complaint.

This is one of the hardest things to grasp initially about homoeopathy but once grasped it makes everything simple. Treat the person, not the disease. Is the person ill in a *Belladonna* way or a *Pulsatilla* way? What helps us to choose the right remedy is the peculiar, personal and distinctive way in which the patient reacts to the illness, the way in which she reacts in the whole of her person and personality: feelings, behaviour, body temperature, appetite, for example.

To be honest, it is not always so easy. Something very marked and acute like earache is likely to be easy to prescribe for because the symptom picture is always clear in a very acute and painful condition like this, as are the changes from the person's normal state. In something more diffused and imprecise like a cold or a headache, where there seem to be a lot of symptoms and none of them are very clear, prescribing may be more difficult.

However, the principle is always the same: try to match as much as possible of the patient's picture in illness to a remedy picture. You should put more emphasis on the general state of the patient than on her particular state, that is, put more emphasis on her general mood, body temperature, appetite, thirst, on the general way she behaves than on the particular named illness from which she appears to be suffering.

What you are looking for is the marked characteristic features of the patient when ill. You then match these to the marked characteristic features of the remedies which you'll find in the *Materia Medica*. Using this approach you will soon realize that some people often need the same remedy whenever they are ill, whatever the precise nature of the named disease, because of their individual and characteristic way of responding to illness, no matter what it is.

When considering the patient's state, it will probably be useful to ask yourself and her or him some of the following questions.

Emotional and Psychological Symptoms

What is her mood like? Is she irritable, tearful, laughing inappropriately, cheerful despite the pain? Is she saying she's fine when she's not? Does she want company, does she want to be alone? Is she quieter than usual? More talkative?

The psychological or emotional picture is extremely important in homoeopathy. It frequently gives us the strongest indications for the remedy, even when the illness seems to be entirely physical. This is not to say that illness is all in the mind, but to acknowledge that emotional and psychological reactions to, or forerunners of, illness are usually very characteristic of the patient and therefore help to individualize the condition more than many other symptoms can.

In acute illness, the psychological response to illness can sometimes show itself in a complete change of character. Mothers often know a child is ill long before a medical symptom appears because they know that she is just 'not herself'. In other cases the emotional nature of the patient may remain the same but become exaggerated. So, for instance, a person who is normally quite shy and reserved might become quite markedly reclusive, taking herself off to her bedroom or being unwilling to go out. What had been just a character trait becomes over-emphasized and more disabling in illness. Either of these types of change is an important symptom.

When a homoeopath treats illness which is long-standing or chronic, she continues to put a lot of emphasis on the psychological or emotional nature of the patient. However, in these cases, the psychological picture will correspond to the way in which the patient normally behaves, and may not be perceived as a symptom or a sign of illness. Our characters, our normal ways of being, our personalities, were not so fixed when we were children; they represent ways of reacting to life emotionally and psychologically which have become hardened, ossified. We wear our life-long characters like coats and think that is who we are, often not noticing that the coat is dirty or out of style, or even that we do not like it any more. In chronic disease a habitual mode of being, a long-established personality pattern is just as much of a symptom as is long-standing joint pain, the typical way someone's digestive system works or the nature of her skin. Homoeopathy will not, of course, change a person's character, but it may help to bring flexibility back into it.

General Physical Symptoms

How is the patient in herself? Is she hot, chilly, sweaty, dry, thirsty, thirstless? Is she unusually hungry or off her food or fancying certain foods, disliking others? Is she over-sensitive to pain or not feeling it enough? Is she drooping around the place or full of frenetic energy? Is she in pain? If so, can she describe the nature of the pains?

These general physical symptoms, states or changes are very important because they affect the whole patient.

Things which make the whole patient feel better or worse are very useful clues: is she better or worse for heat, cold, damp, warmth, fresh air, stuffy rooms, winter, summer, evening, night, morning, 11 a.m., 4 p.m., ice cream?

These physical symptoms, like the psychological symptoms, may have both acute and chronic expressions. In acute disease, which is what you will be treating, look at the changes from the norm; in chronic disease the norm may sometimes be a better guide to the remedy.

Particular Symptoms

These will usually be the symptoms of the actual illness or complaint being suffered. They are things which affect one part of the person. So earache, period pain, colds and joint pain for instance, are all particular symptoms because they can be localized in one part of the patient.

As we've already seen, in homoeopathy these symptoms are less important clues to the remedy than the general symptoms described above, because particular symptoms are usually not very individual with respect to the patient. Particular symptoms are really only of interest when they deviate from what might have been expected, or when they combine with other symptoms in an unusual or characteristic way. There are also particular symptoms which are unusual in themselves, what homoeopaths call strange, rare and peculiar symptoms.

So diarrhoea is one particular symptom: diarrhoea accompanied by a headache makes it a little more specific; joint pain alone is not a very helpful indication for choosing the remedy: joint pain accompanied by indigestion is more individual. An example of a strange, rare and peculiar symptom might be if your complaint was accompanied by a triangular red patch at the tip of the tongue. This symptom is found only in *Rhus tox*. Unfortunately such clear rare symptoms are not very common.

The more unusual the symptom is in connection with the complaint the more important it is. It is not unusual for a cold to be accompanied by a cough, but what might be helpful is the way the patient describes the cough. It might feel as if she has a splinter in her throat (a clue for *Hepar sulph*), or she might hold her ribs when she coughs because she knows the movement will hurt (a clue for *Bryonia*). One patient might get very weepy and clingy with her cold and want to be with people all the time (*Pulsatilla*), another might just disappear to her bedroom and just want to be alone (*Natrum mur*).

These apparently small distinguishing features in every sick person are the important clues, the things that mark this cold as this particular person's cold, not just any cold. No two colds are the same. The nearer you can get to establishing what is different and distinctive about this cold, what is individual about the sufferer's way of having it, the nearer you are to finding the remedy which will relieve it.

In forming a symptom picture the homoeopath will not just rely on what the patient says, but will also note how she says it: whether she is reserved, difficult to get symptoms from: (*Natrum mur, Kali carb*), whether she is outgoing, helpful: (*Phosphorus*), irritable, thinking this is a waste of time: (*Nux vomica*), sceptical but interested, asking questions about the theory of homoeopathy: (*Sulphur*). Is she very anxious about her illness, fearful lest it should be something more serious? (*Arsenicum, Calc carb, Kali carb*). The senses are also used: is there a particular colour of skin? Extreme paleness might indicate *China*, bluey-purple *Lachesis*, red *Sulphur* or *Belladonna*. Is there a particular smell? Sour might indicate *Calc carb*, generally offensive could point to *Sulphur* or *Merc sol*, old cheese might be *Hepar sulph*. All these things are valuable clues.

Having asked all these questions, a professional homoeopath might use a variety of methods to decide on a remedy, consulting books and indexes of symptoms or using a computer system to integrate all the information. If you are doing simpler prescribing for yourself or for your family or friends, then just note down briefly the symptoms which go to make up the patient's symptom picture: the picture of how the patient is when ill. Then put them in an order of importance. A rough guide as to how to grade the symptoms is that the stronger and more obvious a symptom is, the more important it is likely to be; the more spontaneously it is given the more important it is likely to be; the more removed from the patient's normal way of being, the more important it is likely to be. 'Very hot' is better than 'warm' as a symptom. 'Very hot' is an even better symptom if the patient is usually on the chilly side. Important symptoms are also usually those which affect the whole person most. In a long-standing condition they may be the ones which have appeared most recently. Don't worry too much about getting the order right at first: deciding on the relative importance of symptoms is something that comes with practice. Just do it quickly to give yourself a sense of what is important in this patient's picture, where to put the shading or emphasis when you compare it with the remedy picture.

Having formed the symptom picture, you can now begin to try to match it to the picture of a remedy. There are two possible ways of doing that while using this book. One way would be to look up the chapter most likely to include your particular complaint, see which remedies are suggested there for it and then read up the indicated remedies in the *Materia Medica* section to see which best matches the patient in the bigger picture. If the complaint is not particularly specified in any chapter, look it up in the Index of Symptoms at the back of the book and find out from there what remedies may be indicated. Another way would be to look up some of the important general symptoms in the Index of Symptoms and see in what remedies they occur, then follow the same practice of reading through the possible remedy pictures in the *Materia Medica* to see which best matches the whole picture.

Matching the symptom picture of the patient to the symptom picture of the remedy is a skill which develops with practice. In acute illness it is relatively simple to do this, since the disordered symptoms, the symptoms of illness, are usually clear in the person. In chronic illness it is more difficult, since the different layers of symptoms often correspond to the pictures of many different remedies.

Intuition often plays a great part in the selection of the remedy, and once you get used to some of the remedy pictures you will find that it is possible to get a sense of the appropriate remedy long before all the symptoms have been checked. Some very experienced practitioners get a very good idea of the remedy for even chronic disease pictures before they have even begun to ask questions of the patient, because so much can be picked up merely through observation. At first, however, it will be necessary to be more systematic.

Remember that you are not looking for an identical match, only for a remedy picture which is similar to the patient's symptom picture. The stronger the similarity, the greater the likelihood of rapid and complete cure, but it does not have to be a perfect match to work. Remember that in essence what the remedy is doing is stimulating the patient's own immune system to a more vigorous response than it has been capable of until now. Once that has been done, the self-healing system can keep going by itself, at least in the type of illnesses which you will be tackling at first.

Remember, if you choose the wrong remedy nothing will happen. Think again and try another remedy. All you have lost is time.

Chapter Four

CHOOSING THE POTENCY

At this point we need to look briefly at the question of what exactly a remedy is. So far we have been referring to it as if it were precisely the same as the substance from which it is derived. However, by the time we prescribe a remedy in homoeopathic medicine we are no longer using merely a herbal or chemical substance, the plant aconite or the element sulphur for instance: we are also including in our prescription the energetic field around these substances, we are prescribing not aconite itself but the energy of aconite, if you like. This energy is made accessible by the process of preparing the remedies which Hahnemann invented.

When Hahnemann began practising homoeopathy, he was at first concerned only with finding the most similar remedy, and initially prescribed his medicinal substances in the sort of large doses to which he was accustomed from his practice of orthodox medicine. However, since he was now prescribing substances capable of causing the same symptoms as the disease itself had produced in the person he was treating, he soon learned that he needed to give as small a dose as possible in order to avoid overloading the patient's system with symptoms of both disease and drug.

He therefore began to dilute his medicines, and gradually realized that the weaker diluted doses not only had a less damaging impact on the patient, but were actually much more effective in bringing about a cure. Encouraged by this observation, he continued to experiment and discovered that the medicines became even more powerful if they were not only diluted but shaken up vigorously (succussed) during the process of dilution.

He himself thought that the increase in power arose because he had managed to release some of the energy of the substance, some of its spirit, its vital force, as he put it in the language of the eighteenth century. The process and its effects are still far from being fully understood, but it is important to bear in mind that the action of a homoeopathic remedy is dynamic in some way rather than chemical or herbal.

Over a period of years Hahnemann developed a method of diluting and shaking up the remedies in a series designed to regulate the power of his medicines. Briefly, he put a small amount of the medicinal substance into a vial then added 99 parts of a mixture of water and alcohol and shook up the vial: this was called the first dilution: 1. He then took one drop from the resulting liquid, and again added 99 parts of water and alcohol and shook up the vial, this was the second dilution: 2. He took one drop from the resulting liquid, again added 99 parts of water and alcohol and shook up the vial, dilution 3 . . . and so on for as long as his strength lasted.

The more a remedy has been diluted and shaken in this way (potentized), the deeper is its action. So the lower strengths or potencies are less powerful than the higher. Homoeopathic remedies are now available in many different potencies ranging from the 6th, the lowest normally sold, to the CM, or 100,000th. It is best to stay within the lower band of potencies, 6-30, until you get some experience. In fact, many professional homoeopaths rarely prescribe in high potencies.

Most of the remedies included in this book are available in the 6th potency at health food shops and at pharmacies which sell homoeopathic remedies. Some of them are also available in the 30th potency. If you have any difficulty obtaining remedies locally you can order them directly from the manufacturing pharmacies listed in Appendix 2.

With most remedies, and in most conditions, it is probably a good idea to start prescribing with the 6th potency and eventually to move up to the 12th and 30th when you are more confident. In the case of *Aconite, Arnica, Belladonna, Chamomilla* and *Carbo veg* you should buy the 30th potency straight away, because the acute circumstances in which you are likely to use these remedies lend themselves more to the use of the higher potencies. When somebody needs these remedies they usually need as high or as subtle an energy as possible. The lower the potency, the more likely the remedy is to need frequent repetition so if you are prescribing mostly in 6s, 12s or 30s yourself you may have to repeat more often than some homoeopaths who may give you a single remedy in the 10,000th potency (10m) and ask you to come back in a couple of months.

When you have decided what remedy you are going to give your patient and in what potency, give just one dose, or one tablet. Try not to touch the tablet: either tip it from the cap of the bottle into your patient's mouth or tip it into the mouth from a clean piece of paper or a spoon. The patient should then suck the tablet for a few minutes or chew and then suck it if it is very hard. 15-20 minutes should elapse either side of taking a tablet without eating or drinking anything, cleaning teeth or smoking. If you accidentally drop any tablets, throw them away. All these precautions are to protect the remedy from being contaminated by strong smells or tastes or dirt.

If you want homoeopathic remedies to work at their best and if you want to be clear how they work, you should not take other medicines at the same time. However, it is not always possible to be purist about this. *Never* stop taking a prescribed orthodox medicine without consulting your doctor or a health practitioner. It is safe to take homoeopathic remedies at the same time as other medicines and the remedies usually work to some extent in these circumstances, though they are obviously having to work harder, against the flow.

Give the Remedy and Wait

When you have given the remedy, be prepared to wait a while and watch for any reaction. This is the most important instruction to observe in prescribing homoeopathically. Homoeopathic remedies can work extraordinarily quickly: they can also take time to act. The hardest thing is to be patient in prescribing. Be guided by how urgent the situation is. You will find some examples in the next two sections.

It is very difficult to give instructions about how to manage homoeopathic potencies: it is a matter of observation and common sense. In general, remember that you are merely trying to get the body's self-healing system to go into action on its own behalf, not to take over for it. So give the remedy just as much as you need to start this process. Once the process has started do not repeat the remedy until its action has ceased and the patient's improvement stalls or stops. In a long-standing complaint such as joint pain or dyspepsia you may have to repeat the remedy frequently to maintain the improvement. Some specific illustrative examples follow.

Urgent/Acute

If you are trying to stop a haemorrhage or an attack of colic or an earache, then you should expect quick results if you have the right remedy. When the body is in crisis it takes up the remedy very quickly. If you have given the chosen remedy three times in half an hour without any effect, then reconsider the remedy and if it still seems right, then use a higher potency. Start with the 30th potency or the highest you have in these cases. If you think you need a higher potency than the one you have, dissolve a tablet in a glass of water (preferably sterilized or mineral water), and tell your patient to take sips from that, stirring vigorously between each sip. Each sip should be regarded as a dose, and should not be taken till the effect of the last has worn off.

Long-Standing

If, on the other hand, you are treating some long-standing and stubborn condition such as joint pain you should not necessarily expect results until you have taken the remedy, say, twice a day for a week in the 6th potency.

If the improvement is so slight that you can't be sure that it has really taken place, or if your patient is unreliable in her feedback, then repeat the remedy anyway. If the improvement is clear then you can be confident in not repeating the remedy until the symptoms come back . . . and they may not. If there is no response after 3-4 doses in an acute case, or a week in a more chronic case, reconsider the prescription.

Sometimes the use of homoeopathic remedies causes a condition to worsen temporarily before it gets better. This is the aggravation that everyone has heard of in connection with homoeopathy. It is usually quite short-lasting and is accompanied or followed by a general sense of well-being, even though a particular symptom may get temporarily worse. If there is an aggravation, stop and wait for it to settle down before trying the remedy again. (It probably won't happen a second time.)

Aggravations are neither inevitable or necessary. Ideally the aggravation should be short. A headache, for instance, might get briefly worse before it gets better; the patient may feel a little sick or sleepy. The aggravation is normally to some extent proportionate to the strength of the remedy and the illness: that is one reason why it is a good idea to keep to low potencies. Although it may not seem so to the sufferer at the time, an aggravation demonstrates that the body has engaged with the remedy's energy so it is, in fact, usually a good sign. If you are worried at any point, consult a practitioner.

While using homoeopathic remedies it is advisable to avoid strong smells or tastes altogether, especially things like menthol, camphor, peppermint, vapour rubs, aromatic oils, nasal decongestants and strong-flavoured toothpaste. This is because some homoeopaths believe that remedies are antidoted by strong smells and tastes. In any case most of these things are irritants which force the body to do the opposite of what it needs to do, and so are not homoeopathic in themselves. Perhaps it is better to be safe than sorry. It is also possible that drinking coffee may antidote the action of the remedies in some people, so be careful. If your remedies are not working when you think they should be, check to see if the patient is accidentally antidoting them by using strong-smelling or strong-tasting substances.

You can obtain remedies in liquid, granules or tablets. Tablets are probably the most convenient form, and can easily be ground to a powder if you need to give them to a small child. The higher potencies are only used by professional homoeopaths, but you can readily buy some remedies in the 6th and 30th potencies from health food shops or from pharmacies which stock homoeopathic remedies; you can buy other remedies and other potencies by post from manufacturing pharmacists. (See Appendix 2 for details.)

Chapter Five

EMOTIONAL AND
PSYCHOLOGICAL ISSUES

It is becoming more and more difficult to distinguish between psychological, emotional and physical levels of illness. The more we learn, the more it is apparent that the old way of thinking of the body and mind as distinct from each other is no longer useful. Nevertheless, women still suffer from being labelled as neurotic or psychologically ill when they are either being responsive to subtle physical signals of disorder, or expressing themselves emotionally and appropriately. Women are rational beings and we do not need to apologize for the fact that we can also be emotional and sensitive, intuitive and impressionable. In the way that culture and society is currently organized, it is difficult for women to express emotion freely without being labelled as 'over-emotional', 'hysterical' or 'irrational', in Britain at any rate. Women's natural expressions of emotion are often (wrongly) labelled as problems and symptoms by men who are unfamiliar with them and perhaps even disturbed by them. This is bad enough in social relationships, but it is positively dangerous when such judgements are carried over into the medical world.

Homoeopathy treats all parts of the person. As we have seen already in this book, homoeopaths frequently use apparently psychological or emotional symptoms as indications of remedies for apparently physical illnesses. The reverse is also true: physical symptoms can help us confirm the right remedy for an apparently emotional problem. Really, there is no distinction. Illness is a disturbance which expresses itself in various ways in various people at various times; sometimes those ways are called physical, sometimes emotional.

So this chapter is not intended as advice on how to become able to control your feelings 'like a man does'; nor is it intended to show you how to suppress emotions which emerge in response to intolerable situations. Hopefully, what using homoeopathic remedies can do is help you to reach a point of balance where you have a choice about the expression of emotion, and you can choose whether, where and how to express it. You do not have to suppress it, and it is that which is a major cause of illness, both mental and physical.

If at this point you look through the symptoms in the remedies of the *Materia Medica* you will realize that homoeopathy recognizes many different ways or modes of relating to emotions and feelings. There is nothing necessarily 'sick' about any of these. A woman with a *Pulsatilla* constitution will be more inclined to cry openly and to look for support and affection from other people than will a woman with a *Natrum mur* constitution, who will prefer to cry alone on those occasions when she gets in touch with her feelings, and will not express emotions to any but a most trusted friend. A woman with an *Arsenicum* constitution will, in health, deal with her anxiety in a very constructive way, ordering her life and her affairs efficiently in order to remain in a position of choice. A person of a *Phosphorus* or *Arg nit* constitution will, to some extent, rely on the adrenalin rush provided by anxiety, and risk the nervous collapse on the other side of excitement.

We have all developed numerous different ways of relating psychologically to our world. Strictly speaking, of course, all these adaptations are unhealthy because all are defences and stuck positions. However, for most of the time they work well enough.

It is when they do not that we need some help, if the failure of our tried and tested ways of dealing with life is to become a breakthrough to a new way of life rather than a breakdown, or if we are not to get trapped into taking tranquillizers or anti-depressants for long periods. It is at these times that homoeopathic intervention can be invaluable. A remedy can intervene in a process of apparent disintegration sufficiently subtly to let us stand outside what is happening with some calmness, to let us have recovery time, to allow us to make some choices.

Many emotional/psychological problems can be nipped in the bud when they first appear. This is not to say that they should be avoided, or that their usefulness in indicating that something is going wrong should be ignored. I am not advocating the use of homoeopathy to suppress difficult emotions. However, often an emotional reaction to a life event need become no more severe than a physical one. If we take *Arnica* when our bodies are injured, why should we not take *Aconite* or *Staphysagria* when our psyches are injured? It is, after all, only a temporary imbalance. By taking a remedy we can prevent it becoming an all-engulfing problem.

In most cases of emotional stress or strain the body will have been depleted of vitamins and minerals, so it may be useful to take a high-dose multi-vitamin and mineral supplement for a while (take the organic type available from health food shops). B-complex is particularly important because it feeds the nervous system, so take this in addition to the multi-vitamin for a month or so. It may also be helpful to sip *Avena sativa* (wild oat) tincture (available from Galen pharmacy, see Appendix 2) through the day. Dilute half a teaspoonful in a half glass of water. The tissue salt *Kali phos* may be taken daily and the Bach Flower preparation *Rescue Remedy* can be helpful in acute situations. You can obtain these also from your local health food store.

Addiction to Alcohol and Drugs

Addiction to alcohol or drugs often accompanies the chronic suppression of emotion. We drink or take tranquillizers, anti-depressants or so-called recreational drugs to suppress difficult emotions, to enable us to get on with our lives without confronting the issues which are emerging.

Sooner or later comes the decision to try to stop. This is easier said than done. Unless you are very strong-willed, do not attempt to withdraw from drugs, prescribed or otherwise, without the help of an experienced practitioner or counsellor. Sometimes people can be so frightened by the withdrawal effects that they stop withdrawal and never try again. So enter into the process slowly, patiently and with support. Always slow down the rate of withdrawal if you feel panicky. Some people, on the other hand, have no ill-effects beyond mild anxiety or bad temper for a few days.

If insomnia has been part of the problem, use a herbal remedy for sleeplessness to help you over the first difficult weeks and take plenty of calcium and calcium-rich drinks at bed time. Herbal compounds containing passiflora or valerian are helpful and can be obtained from health food stores. (Also see 'Sleeplessness' later in this chapter.)

It will be very helpful to try to adopt a wholefood diet high in complex carbohydrates during any process of withdrawal. The body looks greedily for the nutrients of which it has been depleted, and settles down more quickly if these needs are supplied. Giving in to the temptation to hit the sweets and chocolates for a quick sugar fix draws us into yet another addictive spiral and leads to hypoglycaemia (low blood sugar), with feelings of shakiness and weakness and being unable to cope, and hence back to the drugs and alcohol. For help with a suitable diet, a useful book is Martin Budd's *Low Blood Sugar* (details in Appendix 1).

The following remedies may help both with the effects of the drugs and with the actual withdrawal symptoms.

LACHESIS

This may be useful especially for the effects of alcohol abuse, for the 'social drinker' who gets drunk at parties or in company, is scintillatingly witty and entertaining or feels angry and persecuted and can't remember a word that was said the next morning.

NUX VOMICA

This is always the first remedy to consider in any question of drug or alcohol dependency. The general picture of the remedy corresponds very well to that of the addiction-prone personality: it contains the whole spiral of addiction including the liver damage. It is also most useful in helping moderate the anxiety, panic, irritability and muscle spasm often associated with withdrawal.

SULPHUR

This is a great cleansing remedy. It may be useful where there has been solitary drinking and nervous exhaustion has set in. Use *Nux vomica* during the process of withdrawal, *Sulphur* after withdrawal is completed.

The following remedies may help with some of the specific withdrawal symptoms:

Aconite: Sudden panic, fear of dying, feeling chilly.
Arnica: Bruised sore sensations.
Arsenicum: Great anxiety, restlessness, fear of being alone.
Rhus tox: Muscle stiffness and soreness.

Anxiety and Fear

Acute anxiety and fear cannot easily be distinguished. They bring on the same frightening physical symptoms: palpitations, pains around the heart, shallow rapid breathing (hyperventilation), even numbness and tingling in the fingers and toes. The sufferer may wake in the middle of the night in a panic and may not be able to go back to sleep. The reason for the anxiety is often clear: it is entirely appropriate to react with anxiety, fear, and panic to a shattering life event: an accident involving friends or family, a car crash, a death, a threat of separation or other such events. Sometimes there is no readily apparent explanation and the attack may be triggered by something having stirred up an unconscious association from the past, as in some phobias, for instance. At other times the cause may lie in a nervous system made over-sensitive and over-reactive from continued stress.

Chronic anxiety will produce similar symptoms in a milder or more sporadic way. The root cause here is often buried in childhood. Working with a counsellor may help you to identify the nature and origins of particular patterns of reaction that may no longer be necessary but which have become habitual. These reactive patterns carry feelings with them from a much earlier time in your life when you were unable to act to solve the problem you faced. Homoeopathic treatment can also intervene and help shift these patterns. Sometimes a remedy will lift the anxiety just enough to make it possible to risk talking about it to someone else.

Anxiety takes many forms, but is usually part of a web of defences against total panic. When we suffer from phobias we become afraid of specific situations. This is usually a creative attempt by the organism to localize free-floating anxiety and fear so that we can actually continue our lives. In many ways it is very efficient to maintain a localized fear of mice, birds, snakes or spiders. These are things which can usually be avoided in life.

However, problems arise when such fears are localized onto something which cannot be avoided: for example, claustrophobia which prevents people from using lifts, cars, or underground transport systems, or shopping in department stores, or agoraphobia, which stops people from going outside their houses at all.

The following remedies may be indicated. You can look them up in more detail in the *Materia Medica*. Other remedies also include anxiety in their picture, and references to these may be found in the Index.

ACONITE

In acute attacks, where there is panic, palpitations, restlessness, shallow breathing, agitation and sensations of numbness and tingling. It is useful in panic attacks, agoraphobia, claustrophobia and emotional shock.

ARGENTUM NITRICUM

This kind of state is hurried and dithery. The person rushes about with anxiety, everything has to happen in a hurry, and so it doesn't happen properly. They can't settle down, like the White Rabbit from *Alice in Wonderland*. There is strong anticipatory anxiety and the sufferer will be hurried and flustered, possibly even trembling and suffering from nervous diarrhoea.

ARSENICUM

This is indicated in chronic anxiety, in the perpetual worrier, especially where the anxiety centres on getting things right or keeping things in order, or where there is anxiety about time, meeting deadlines or appointments, an inability to be late. The anxiety may be accompanied by breathlessness, palpitations and a feeling of chilliness.

CAUSTICUM

This is indicated in a chronically timid and anxious woman, often an older woman with a frail constitution, where physical weakness and an over-sensitive nervous system contributes to the development of fears. A cautious anxiety is characteristic: anxiety with fear that something will happen; she is fearful of her own thoughts, easily startled. She has a particular fear of the dark.

GELSEMIUM
A remedy for acute anticipatory anxiety, exam nerves, school phobia. Fear will bring about a near paralysis, legs will go like jelly and the person will be unable to remember a thing. May have diarrhoea.

LYCOPODIUM
This remedy is indicated where there is chronic anxiety of anticipation and fear of failure, which may be concealed and controlled until the woman needs to give a speech, give a performance, take an exam or otherwise expose herself to criticism. She will overprepare then perform very well or achieve excellent results, but will still feel inadequate and lack self-confidence. She may assume an air of superiority to mask her fear. Fear of change, of anything new is also marked.

PHOSPHORUS
This is often useful in sensitive, imaginative people who fear the dark, shadows, ghosts. They are afraid that something might happen, they do not know what. They are terrified of thunderstorms. They are worse at twilight and need constant reassurance.

PULSATILLA
This remedy is indicated for nervous timid people who need a lot of reassurance. They will suffer from claustrophobia in stuffy rooms, fear of being alone, of the dark, of ghosts in the evening, of crowds. They are likely to be irritable when anxious. They worry about whether other people approve of them.

SILICA
This is indicated in shy and timid people who have a great fear of undertaking things, fear that they will fail, but also have a dogged determination to succeed once anything has been undertaken.

Bereavement/Grief

Grief is not an illness, and it can indeed eventually prove a point of growth: it is, however, a very lonely state. It is also an extremely difficult state to manage, including as it might despair, guilt, anger, terror, feelings of one's own mortality and an almost obsessional tendency to recall the lost person. Sometimes it is too difficult to grieve, and we just cut off from the whole process. We go underground and pretend we are all right; indeed, we believe that we should be. Our culture supports this. Even the well-meaning attempts to help us grieve, which talk of stages and times of mourning, may make us feel we are doing it wrong when we find that everything happens in confusion and we don't meet the milestones. The remedies indicated below will not suppress grief, they will not make it go away; they will, however, encourage and allow the process to unfold in whatever way the individual mourner needs.

ACONITE
This may be indicated in cases of sudden death where shock and panic are uppermost.

CAUSTICUM
People who need *Causticum* are extremely sympathetic to others and may grieve as much for the others as for themselves. It may be particularly indicated where anxiety and confusion follow bereavement.

IGNATIA
This remedy contains all the contradictions of the grieving state in its picture: there is a mixture of sighs, tears and laughter, anger, anxiety, fear and extravagant expression of emotion side by side with a silent sadness which cannot be expressed.

NATRUM MUR

This is indicated when grief has been binding someone for many years. There is a strong sense of having had something very precious stolen from them and they cannot let it go from their memory.

PULSATILLA

This is indicated where grief is unexpressed in a normally emotionally expressive person. Loss, particularly of an important family member, is devastating for the *Pulsatilla* type who needs constant support and reassurance.

STAPHYSAGRIA

This may be useful in a reserved grief where the bereaved person has difficulty in experiencing or expressing the anger associated with loss.

Depression

Depression is a word that covers a multitude of states. What they have in common is a weary, flat attitude to life, which no longer feels worth living. There may be thoughts of suicide. The sufferer feels cut off from everyone else, feels a failure and is often impossible to reach emotionally, especially by family members. Deep depression is a serious and terrible state to be in, and the sufferer will need a lot of help and support to move out of it.

It used to be thought that there were two types of depression, endogenous (caused by chemical change) and reactive (caused by events, life). This no longer seems to be the predominant theory. Usually depression is due to complex psychological processes which need to be unravelled before a real cure can take place. Remedies will often aid the recall of forgotten causal events.

Women frequently suffer from transient depression related to the shift of hormones. Some depression is undoubtedly caused by poor nutrition. If the body is deprived of the vitamins it needs, especially the B range, then a woman can feel exhausted and depressed. The following remedies reflect some of the different ways in which depression can be expressed.

ARSENICUM

This is a restless sort of depression, depression in its agitated anxious, obsessional form, the sufferer is full of self-reproach. Guilt is the predominant expression of the state. She thinks she has offended her friends and that they hate her. She is also frequently highly critical of others.

CIMICIFUGA

The woman feels as though a black cloud is hanging over her. She feels that people want to kill her, poison her. This severe depression is often associated with childbirth, when she may even wish the child harm. There may be sudden unpredictable bouts of depression.

LACHESIS

An intense depression often following loss, failure of an enterprise, personal rejection. It can also be associated with the menopause and with any time when there is loss of sexual libido.

NATRUM MUR

This covers a really deep depressive state, often too deep for the sufferer to acknowledge fully. She bottles up emotions and rejects sympathy because it is 'false' or embarrasses her. She prefers to be alone and avoids company.

NUX VOMICA

It is sometimes difficult to see the depression in this remedy because the subject is more inclined to anger and blame of others than of self. However, this behaviour is often a defence against self-blame and when it fails, the person can flip over into severe depression mixed with anger and indignation. The trigger for depression may be humiliation arising from the failure of some enterprise.

SEPIA

A very deeply depressed state is represented in this remedy. There is no interest in anything: family, friends, work, sexual activity. The woman just 'can't be bothered' with any of the things in which she would normally be highly involved and active. Whatever is suggested will be criticized. The depression is often precipitated by overwork and adrenal exhaustion. It may also follow viral infection or childbirth.

Eating Disorders

Dieting and compulsive eating seem to be emotional issues for most women during at least some period of our lives. Some of the reasons seem to lie in a complex response to our position as objects of sexual admiration and rejection over thousands of years. If we are lucky, such considerations only affect our eating habits transiently, at times when we feel particularly personally vulnerable, low in self-esteem. Some women, however, get caught in a vicious and guilty cycle of bingeing and dieting which takes over their lives. Bulimia and anorexia, the extreme forms of these two compulsions, can even threaten life. If you suspect these in yourself or your family you should make every effort to get experienced help. The following remedies may prove useful adjuncts to professional therapy.

ARSENICUM

The desire for control over self and the environment is one of the strongest characteristics of the *Arsenicum* personality, and it is such a person who is most prone to develop an over-controlling self-punishing relationship to food and health. She tends to be naturally thin and a quick metabolizer of food; at times she cannot stand the sight or smell of it.

CALCAREA CARBONICA

A person of this remedy type can become anorexic from feeling inadequate. A natural weight-gainer, she may eat voraciously and pile on even more weight to protect further her vulnerable inner self, or may be tempted to overeat and then induce vomiting.

NATRUM MUR

This kind of person finds it difficult to express feelings directly and is therefore at risk of expressing them through comfort eating or rejection of food. She can either crave or hate bread and salt, two foods symbolically associated with life itself.

SULPHUR

This remedy has an excessive appetite and a constant craving for food, especially sweet food. It is very useful in bulimic eating.

Sleeplessness/Insomnia

There are many remedies with sleeplessness in their picture: it is, however, always only a part of the larger picture which should be looked at carefully in prescribing.

The following remedies may be of use in acute or transient sleeplessness:

Aconite: after shock or panic, with restlessness, nightmares, fear of dying.

Arnica: when too tired to sleep, fidgety, bed feels too hard.

Arsenicum: when waking between midnight and 2 a.m. restless, worried, apprehensive and possibly with foreboding dreams of fire or danger.

Chamomilla: especially for children who are wide awake and irritable in the early part of the night and want to be carried.

Coffea: where the mind is overactive, inability to switch off.

Lycopodium: mind is very active at bedtime, going over and over work done during day; dreams a lot, talks and laughs in sleep. Wakes around 4 a.m.

Nux vomica: sleeplessness as a result of great mental strain, overindulgence in food or alcohol or withdrawal from alcohol or sleeping tablets. Person wakes around 3 or 4 a.m. and then falls asleep just as it is time to get up.

Rhus tox: restless, walks about, especially if there is pain or discomfort.

This chapter has only uncovered the tip of the iceberg of emotional states in which homoeopathy can help to restore balance and choice. In the hands of skilled practitioners, homoeopathy is capable of bringing enormous relief and clarity to people who suffer from psychological problems of various kinds, and my hope is that by using some of the remedies indicated above you will obtain short-term help of a kind which will open up to you the potential of homoeopathy in this field.

Chapter Six

MENSTRUATION

The experience of being a woman is completely different from the experience of being a man. Although this may seem an obvious statement, it is something that is largely ignored even in this modern liberated age. We live in a society where one of the most fundamental of women's experiences, the emotional fluctuation caused by hormonal changes within the body throughout the month, is more or less completely unacknowledged, accepted only when it can be used to make allowances for women's 'strange' behaviour. 'Her period must be due' is regarded as explanation and excuse for what is often justified anger in women.

Menstruation is prominent in a woman's life for a very long time and yet the whole process is still shrouded in secrecy, mystery and even shame. Even though sex is talked about freely in the pages of women's magazines, bleeding is not so popular. It is only fairly recently that much public acknowledgment has been given to it. Up till now we have had to wonder in secret about whether we bleed heavily or not (what is heavy bleeding?); about whether we should be getting the amount of pain we get; about whether we need to be as unhappy and irritable as we sometimes are before periods.

Menstruation is not an illness but a natural process. However, like other natural processes, its efficient working can be interrupted by a variety of causes. Anxiety, stress, grief, travel, swimming or even getting your feet wet, taking the Pill or being ill in some way can all upset the delicate hormonal balance, and in these situations homoeopathy can intervene to restore it. Obviously, repeated or chronic difficulties with periods are the province of chronic treatment and should be attended to by an experienced homoeopath. Within the larger picture, however, there are many symptoms which may well be amenable to acute treatment, for instance transient period pains, heavy bleeding and sore breasts. This chapter is intended more to show the potential of homoeopathy in this important area of life than to suggest extensive self-treatment.

During the years of menstruation it is important to use tampons and the Pill as sparingly as possible. The Pill has been the subject of a good deal of controversy, and there is no reason to think that this is at an end. It has been implicated in many cases of erosion of the cervix, cervical cancer, breast cancer and circulatory problems. Despite adjustments to the level of the hormones and steroids involved, there still seems to be an unnecessarily high risk to health associated with the use of the Pill. As for tampons, they are so absorbent that they cause dryness in the vagina and roughen the vaginal walls, thus increasing the vulnerability to infections. The chlorine with which they are bleached is also an irritant.

Puberty

The beginning of menstruation can be a very difficult time. When it is delayed there can be a lot of embarrassment, especially if it is associated with a general delayed development of breasts and pubic hair, so visible in the school changing room. Everyone develops in their own time, but there are homoeopathic remedies which may put a sluggish system into gear a little more quickly.

The major remedy for disturbances in the onset and

establishment of menstruation is *Pulsatilla*. With its picture of changeability, easy emotion, tearfulness and irritability, it corresponds very well to the difficult state young girls may get into when their periods are not established, including the 'stomach migraine' that sometimes appears before the beginning of menstruation. *Natrum muriaticum* is also very strongly indicated for menstruation delayed into the late teens. If the girl has been a little slow in her general physical development then *Calc carb* or *Silica* might be considered.

Amenorrhoea (Absence of Periods)

Sometimes, once established, menstruation then stops. Often this is due to nerves, fatigue, travel, or some other environmental factor. It is also associated with overtraining in sportswomen, loss of body fat and anorexia. *Pulsatilla* is again likely to be the first remedy to consider, followed by *Calc carb* and *Nat mur*. If the interruption to the cycle is the result of shock or cold consider *Aconite*; if of grief or some other emotional upset consider *Ignatia*, or *Nat mur*. *Nat mur* is particularly strongly indicated if there has been long-standing emotional upset.

Pre-Menstrual Syndrome

Once menstruation has established itself most women have at least some times when they regret its existence. PMS or pre-menstrual syndrome is a reality. I am constantly amazed by how many women apologetically say that yes, they feel worse before a period but that it is (a) to be expected and (b) all in the mind anyway. No one who has ever experienced the sharp change in mood and sense of self that sometimes comes on before a period can deny that there is a change, and that it is not in any way self-induced. Many women can feel the precise moment of change inside their bodies, a sudden descent into a pit of depression or an explosion into anger which is absolutely and qualitatively different from other kinds of depression or anger.

This is also a time when suppressed emotion leaks out. A woman may say 'I'm not myself' but she probably means 'I'm not the self I've been pretending to be'. It is a time when the normal woman's capacity to suppress anger and other feelings and dreams and get on with the practicalities of life may be suspended. In the grip of the hormonal disturbance, the suppressed resentments of the years may come flooding out, especially in a woman of a *Nat mur* type. Sometimes this is to the good. However, if you do not want to be at the mercy of your hormones, if you do not want to feel the effects of their imbalance for ten days a month, read on. It does not need to happen. You do not need to feel out of control as well as unable to express anger and distress. If you are able to control the hormonal imbalance, you may well find a more effective way to express whatever substantial feelings remain.

PMS is, of course, often a deep-seated problem and should be treated by an experienced homoeopath. But if there is none in your area, try one of the following remedies on an acute basis and see what kind of relief you get. Although it is the emotional symptoms which are most talked about because of their effects in the home and at work, PMS usually also includes some tenderness of the breasts, general fluid retention leading to increase in weight, slight abdominal distension and twinges of pain. These symptoms, however, tend to be common to a number of remedies and it is within the range of the psychological symptoms that you are most likely to find those which characterize the particular remedy you may need.

Calc carb, Lachesis, Natrum muriaticum, Nux vomica, Pulsatilla and *Sepia* all have the common physical and emotional symptoms of PMS.

CALC CARB

The timidity, nervousness and self-consciousness of *Calc carb* may well be emphasized at these times, as well as her craving for eggs and sweet things.

LACHESIS

In this remedy all symptoms will be worse in the morning after sleep, worse for wearing tight clothing and will improve dramatically as soon as the bleeding starts.

NAT MUR

The woman will be irritable and unwilling to talk to anyone, will just want to be by herself. Fluid retention will be marked and there may be migraines for this reason.

NUX VOMICA

The woman will be irritable and angry, still trying to get everything done faster but with less energy. She may be constipated and crave sweet or fatty foods.

PULSATILLA

The woman will be markedly irritable, touchy and weepy, needing constant company, attention and reassurance. She might also feel nauseous with fainting, back pain and headaches. She'll be much worse for stuffy rooms at these times, positively claustrophobic, and much better in the open air.

SEPIA

The woman, though every bit as irritable and angry as *Nux vom*, even to the point of wanting to run away from home and never see the family again, will be much more depressed. She will be absolutely unwilling to eat fatty foods, craving sweet or salty foods, and will be totally uninterested in any sexual relationship.

Other remedies to consider, if the general symptoms agree, may be *Arsenicum, Causticum, Cimicifuga, Kali carb, Lycopodium, Sulphur*.

Period Pains (Dysmenorrhoea)

The period itself can be extremely painful. Women tend to expect pain during a period, it's part of our mythology, but it is not inevitable. There should be no more than mild and transient discomfort associated with the time of bleeding.

The following remedies may be considered:

BELLADONNA
Extremely heavy and violently painful periods with bright red clotted blood. There is an aching dragging sensation made worse by lying down. The woman will be hot with a red face, and very sensitive to movement.

CAULOPHYLLUM
This has severe cramping labour-like pains, better when the bleeding starts (though not as dramatically better as is *Lachesis*).

CHAMOMILLA
This has severe, colicky, labour-like pains. Vomiting and diarrhoea are common. The woman gets very angry and is extremely intolerant of noise and pain.

CIMICIFUGA
The sufferer has to double over with sharp labour-like pains that dart from side to side in the abdomen. There is marked lower-back pain during the flow and the pain is worse for movement.

COLOCYNTHIS
The pain is relieved by doubling up, pressure, warmth. The woman

is irritable and angry. Pains can come on after or with suppression of anger.

IPECAC
Heavy periods where the bleeding amounts to haemorrhaging: the pain will probably be accompanied by nausea.

LACHESIS
The pain will be severe and congestive, probably accompanied by a headache; it will be bad before the flow is established and improve rapidly once the bleeding starts. There may also be pain in the small of the back or dizziness before menstruation. Pains tend to be worse on the left side, around the ovary. Cannot bear tight clothing.

NUX VOMICA
The pain is characteristically cramping and spasmodic with a tendency to low back pain. Irritability and spasms of anger will be marked. Periods are often early and prolonged and there my be constipation and bladder irritation.

PULSATILLA
The cutting tearing pains may be accompanied by nausea and vomiting as well as weepiness. Periods are usually late and slight.

SEPIA
The chief characteristic symptom is the sagging, dragging feeling, the sensation that her insides will fall out. Nausea, low back pain and a deep despair may accompany the pains. Periods tend to be irregular.

Evening Primrose Oil, Calcium and Magnesium supplements have also proved helpful in some cases, as well as Vitamin B6. Do not take B6 in isolation from other vitamins of the B range.

Breast Problems

Of course, our breasts also respond quickly to hormonal changes. Many of us don't even like to think about breasts. Any kind of pain and tenderness in that area seems to strike terror in us. Go straight to your health practitioner if you have any worrying suspicions. In the unlikely event that you do have a malignancy, the sooner it is detected the better, no matter what form of treatment you may choose. You can also easily learn how to examine your breasts for yourself either from a book such as *Our Bodies Ourselves* (see Appendix 1), from a Well Woman clinic, or from your doctor.

Most changes and lumps in the breast have less frightening causes. It is quite normal for breasts to feel slightly tender before periods. The glands in the breast can also swell, as they can anywhere else when the body is fighting general infection of any kind. Benign cysts (fluid-filled sacs of tissue) and fibroadenosis, thickening of glandular tissue for no known reason, are also common.

The remedies most likely to be useful in uncomplicated breast tenderness before periods are *Phytolacca* and *Pulsatilla*.

PHYTOLACCA
The glands in the armpits may be swollen and the woman may feel shivery. There may be a purplish tinge to the breast which may feel particularly tender before and during a period. Characteristically there will be stony hard nodules with shooting pains. The problem may be associated with cold damp weather or emotional strain.

PULSATILLA
The notable feature of *Pulsatilla* breast pain is that the pain comes and goes suddenly, reducing the woman to tears. There may be milk in the breasts at times. The woman is likely to feel hot and uncomfortable, weepy and irritable.

Thrush and Cystitis

Embarrassing 'female' problems are also intimately connected with the process of menstruation and hormonal change. Itching (pruritus) and catarrhal discharges of various origins (leucorrhoea) are common at this time. The dreaded thrush and cystitis are often worse before periods. Women are unfortunate in that the openings of vagina, bladder and anus are all very close together which makes it easy for infection to spread from one to the other.

Cystitis is something many women suffer from, often after sex, which makes them dread it. Something like 75 per cent of women suffer from vaginal thrush at some point in their lives and almost 100 per cent from pruritus, coyly referred to as 'feminine itching' in adverts for ointments aimed at relieving it. So you are not alone, and there is nothing to be ashamed about.

A lot of the itching and inflammation is the result of irritation arising from the use of various creams, bath salts and foam, soaps, deodorants, talcum powder and washing powder. It can be caused by tampons, sanitary towels, vigorous sex, contraceptives, too-tight clothing, cycling. Check all of these; even if you have been using one of them for a long time without ill effects, sensitivities and allergies can develop at any time.

THRUSH

Thrush seems to be the most prevalent problem of them all. We are nearly all going to have it, or suspect that we have it, at some time in our life. We are becoming more and more aware that *Candida albicans*, the yeast that causes thrush, has colonized more and more of us. Vaginal thrush, embarrassing as it is, is merely the tip of the iceberg. *Candida* is everywhere, and it loves the modern diet of sugar and yeast-based foods. If you have it you may get a rash on your body or recurrent tiredness, bloatedness, depression, food cravings, digestive problems and sore throats. If you have it in the vagina you'll probably notice itchiness and soreness and a thick white discharge looking a bit like cottage cheese and smelling a bit like newly-baked bread. Urination will be more frequent than usual and there will be some slight stinging.

Women often feel quite desperate in the face of these stubborn and recurring infections. However, they can only develop if acid-producing bacteria in the vagina have been destroyed, so the first thing to do is to restore the acid environment of the vagina by, for example, using a vinegar and water douche or a garlic suppository. Some women find it helpful to insert live yogurt or Aloe Vera gel (available in many pharmacies/health/cosmetic shops) into the vagina for a few nights.

You can cut down on sugar and yeast products in your diet (cut them out, even, for a short time) or, if the condition is severe, follow a strict anti-*Candida* diet, though this can sometimes increase sensitivity to food. And you can approach the problem homoeopathically. The best indicated homoeopathic remedies are, if the general picture agrees with that of the patient: *Pulsatilla, Sepia* and *Borax*.

PULSATILLA

This is probably the most useful remedy since its general catarrhal condition and characteristic yellow or yellow-green, creamy, bland (sometimes irritating) discharge corresponds so exactly to the symptoms. In addition, the condition is common just before periods when a woman is most likely to be in a *Pulsatilla* state. The remedy is well indicated for vaginal inflammation and itching during pregnancy and in girls during puberty. The condition, as usual with *Pulsatilla*, will be worse in the evening, lying down and in hot stuffy conditions.

SEPIA

This will be useful where the yellow/green discharge is more smarting and offensive than that of *Pulsatilla* and is likely to be worse in the morning and while walking. Constipation, irritability and exhaustion are marked.

BORAX

This is almost a specific for thrush, whether vaginal or in the mouth. Use it when the vaginal discharge is clear and thick like the white of an egg or liquid starch. The discharge may be bland or irritating and be accompanied by a sensation like warm water; it is sometimes worse in the middle of the menstrual cycle.

Arsenicum, Calc carb and *Merc sol* may also be considered if the symptoms match. *Sulphur* may be useful in chronic problems.

CYSTITIS

Cystitis is intricately linked to thrush, largely because the standard orthodox medical treatment for cystitis is antibiotics, which cause thrush by destroying the friendly bacteria in the bowel and allowing the *Candida* to spread unchecked. Women can easily get locked into a vicious cycle of thrush and cystitis. Fifteen per cent of adult women get repeated attacks of cystitis, and it is even more common in late pregnancy.

Common symptoms are burning pain during urination, frequent and powerful urging to urinate though little urine may be passed, and cloudy or bloody urine. Pain or tenderness in the lower abdomen or the back, fever and a feeling of being generally ill may also accompany cystitis. There are several ways of keeping this complaint at bay. The primary one, of course, is to be very hygienic. Always wash carefully (preferably without soap, which can be an irritant), and avoid tight clothing around this area. If there is an actual attack, drink a lot of water to cleanse the kidneys.

The following remedies all include in their picture the basic symptoms of cystitis. The distinguishing and characteristic symptoms of each remedy will give an accurate match to the way in which each woman individually experiences cystitis. Check in the fuller *Materia Medica* to see whether the remedy fits the whole of the patient's picture. These remedies would be useful to check an acute attack of cystitis, but if the condition is chronic with recurring attacks, the advice of a professional homoeopath should be sought.

ACONITE

This will be indicated in the earliest stages, when burning sensations on urinating are first noticed. If taken soon enough, it may stop other symptoms from developing.

CANTHARIS

This is the remedy for the worst attacks of cystitis, and will usually help to some degree in any case. There will be very strong burning, cutting, stabbing pains in the lower abdomen, before, during and after urination, along with a very strong, almost continuous urging to urinate, even just after doing so. The patient will be bad-tempered, restless and even frantic with the severe pain. Sexual desire may be increased. Intensity and rapidity mark this remedy.

Apis and *Arsenicum* are quite hard to distinguish from *Cantharis* in cystitis but *Cantharis* will be much more violent in its symptoms.

APIS

You may need *Apis* where the pains are worse for heat and at night and better for cold, the patient is restless and anxious and the abdomen is sensitive to the slightest touch. The sufferer will be thirstless.

ARSENICUM ALBUM
The sufferer will be very restless but chilly, anxious and very thirsty for frequent short cold drinks. The marked burning pains will be better for heat and warmth.

CAUSTICUM
This may be helpful where the condition affects older women. There is a frequent urge to pass urine, made worse by coughing or sneezing, along with an acute sensitivity to cold. The woman will go to the toilet in response to an urge, fail to produce any urine and then soon afterwards lose urine involuntarily.

MERC SOL
This has all the typical symptoms of cystitis and is characterized by being one of the few remedies indicated when the burning pain is worse when the patient is not urinating.

STAPHYSAGRIA
This should be considered when an attack comes on after sexual intercourse, catheterization or rape, attempted rape, any form of sexual abuse. The pains are typically sharp and cutting.

Chapter Seven

PREGNANCY AND LABOUR

Homoeopathy can be of great help in all the circumstances surrounding conception, pregnancy, labour and the early days after having your child. It is clearly a good idea to consult a homoeopathic practitioner as soon as you know you want a baby. Then if there are any difficulties in conception caused by hormone imbalance, the remedies may be able to help overcome these without the need for strong drug therapy. Nutritional deficiencies can also be responsible for a failure to conceive: a combination of remedies and supplements may change the picture.

Once you are pregnant it is even more important that you should be under the guidance of a practitioner. Pregnancy is not, of course, an illness; however, there are discomforts and imbalances which can occur during it which can be adjusted in order to make the process easier. Some of these things are definitely the province of an experienced practitioner: conditions such as threatened miscarriage and high blood pressure. If the baby is in a bad position in the womb, it can often be turned by the use of appropriate homoeopathic remedies. Usually a homoeopathic practitioner will be glad to work in conjunction with you and your doctor, to make sure you get all the support you need. Homoeopathic remedies have never been suspected of causing any problems in pregnancy, and it is just as safe to be treated homoeopathically for coughs, colds and other conditions at this time as at any other. Ideally, you should not treat either yourself or anyone else during pregnancy unless you are a qualified homoeopath. This section has been included to give you some sense of what is treatable, and what you might do for yourself or in consultation with your homoeopath.

The following conditions are particularly likely to arise.

Backache

Sepia is well-indicated for the general sagging condition of all the muscles and internal organs, especially if the woman is exhausted and harassed.

Arnica and *Rhus tox* may be considered if the backache is regarded as an injury or strain caused by carrying the baby or moving awkwardly.

Kali carb is perhaps the major remedy to be considered in this kind of backache due to weakened ligaments. Use it especially if extremely weak and tired, sweating easily and with digestive problems.

Constipation

Nux vomica is the first remedy to think of, if the irritability and drive characteristic of it is present.

Sepia is also indicated, but would present a more tired and lethargic picture.

Bryonia might be considered if the stool is very dry and the woman very thirsty and irritable, especially if there is also muscle and joint pain worse for movement.

Emergencies

Serious emergencies can obviously arise during a pregnancy, and if you suspect a threatened miscarriage or an ectopic pregnancy you should arrange for medical assistance immediately. However, while waiting for help the following may be useful:

Aconite, if there is great fear and anxiety.

Arnica, if there has been a fall or injury or if abdominal pain is involved.

Ipecac or *Belladonna* may help if given frequently in the case of heavy bleeding or haemorrhaging.

If you have a history of miscarriage please consult a practitioner, as there are remedies which can assist in this problem.

Heartburn/Indigestion

This is often a problem late in the pregnancy when the womb is pressing on the digestive system.

Nux vomica might be the first remedy to think of where the general symptoms agree: chilliness, irritability and a disposition to hard work should be present.

Pulsatilla may be indicated if the problem arises after rich or fatty foods, and where the woman is inclined to be tearful and feel helpless.

China may be indicated especially where there is a lot of flatulence and bloating.

Morning Sickness

This is most common in the 5th-12th weeks of pregnancy and can actually be present at any time of the day. It is a strongly characteristic symptom of the following remedies:

Ipecacuanha will relieve most cases temporarily, and is especially indicated where the nausea is accompanied by irritability, a dry cough or a tendency to easy bleeding, nose bleeds.

Kali carb is a remedy where anxiety especially affects the stomach and should be considered where there is sweating, weakness and a general tendency to water retention. There may be waves of nausea.

Sepia is well-indicated where there is a general state of exhaustion. The nausea is likely to be constant but worse 3-5 p.m. The woman feels better for eating but doesn't want to eat.

Arsenicum may be useful if the general picture agrees. Extreme anxiety about own and child's health is likely to be present.

Morning sickness may be due to a shortage of vitamin B6, and in mild cases extra B vitamins may be all that is needed. In other cases taking care to eat small amounts of protein (e.g. cheese, eggs, tofu, fish, nuts) at regular (2-hour) intervals through the day will prevent low blood sugar from developing and with it the nausea.

Piles and Varicose Veins

Hamamelis is indicated very strongly in the treatment of women with varicose veins and piles, especially the sort of piles that occur towards the end of the pregnancy and after the birth.

Pulsatilla or *Nux vomica* may also be indicated where the general symptoms agree.

Nelson's make a Pile Ointment which can offer some relief.

Miscarriage

If you miscarry, allow yourself to grieve. In the rush of the practical details you may feel that it is not all right to grieve, or that it is just one of those things. Follow how your body feels, and allow the loss.

Similarly, if for any reason you need an abortion, do not neglect or try to suppress your feelings. Even if it was the best thing to do, and on balance you have no regrets, that is only one part of you speaking. Another part needs help to grieve.

Aconite or *Ignatia* may help you get over the shock to the system and the feelings of loss, and your practitioner will be able to give remedies which will help in drying up the milk supply.

Labour

Caulophyllum is extremely useful in childbirth. Period pains and pains in the small joints are also strongly represented in its picture. A general lack of muscular tone is characteristic.

It will be useful when it is difficult to establish labour, when the contractions are short and irregular, or when they stop altogether. The cervix will be rigid and will not dilate. The pains will be spasmodic and flit around; the woman will feel chilly.

In general it may be particularly helpful at the contractions stage: dissolve a tablet in a glass of water and sip from the glass from time to time, or whenever you feel a contraction to be imminent. Some homoeopaths suggest taking one tablet daily for the last few days before the labour starts, but it seems preferable to wait for the symptoms to appear.

Kali carb may be helpful if the characteristic stitching jerking pains are present and if the difficulty is due to weakness.

Pulsatilla and *Cimicifuga* may also be useful.

After the Birth

Arnica is invaluable for the bruising and soreness inevitable after childbirth.

Staphysagria will be particularly important if the birth has been difficult and has required a lot of intervention, especially after an episiotomy, or if the woman feels humiliated that she has not been allowed to have the baby 'naturally'.

Kali carb is one of the best remedies for the after-effects of childbirth, especially where there is great weakness and stitching afterpains flitting around the body.

Breastfeeding

If there is not enough milk to feed the baby, consider *Agnus castus*. This is indicated when the milk supply has eased as soon as it has started, and the woman becomes weak and exhausted. *Phytolacca* will also be strongly indicated in such cases.

If these fail then consider *Pulsatilla* or *Causticum*. (Certain Irish brands of stout are said to be wonderful, as well as fennel tea.)

Urtica is indicated where there is a complete absence of milk along with stinging nettle-like pains.

If there is a complete aversion to breastfeeding, then consider *Sepia*.

Sore Cracked Nipples

Calendula ointment applied externally will bring considerable relief. *Calendula* tablets may also be taken internally to help prevent infection.

Possible complications following damage to the nipples are mastitis and even breast abscesses.

Aconite taken at the first sign of trouble may help, but if the condition develops then *Phytolacca* is the first remedy to consider.

Here the breast is usually very hard but tender and inflamed. There is a combination of backache, shivering and a raised temperature. Often the left breast is worse.

Bryonia and *Belladonna* may also be useful.

Hot and cold compresses may be applied.

If these measures do not bring relief, consult a practitioner.

Post-Natal Depression

This can occur at anytime in the first year after the birth. The first thing to say is that you should not put up with it, and you should not blame yourself. At the time of birth there is a huge drop in the hormone level, which in itself can cause depression. You have also just been through a long period of hard physical work; you may have had a difficult labour. Some degree of hormonal and emotional let down is to be expected, even if the baby is the best thing that ever happened to you. Through the first year after the birth the hormones remain out of kilter, and your energy may be depleted by breast-feeding, broken nights and the generally very tiring procedure of being responsible for a demanding and helpless human being for 24 hours a day. It is quite natural to feel stressed, depressed and unable to cope.

You will be more likely to feel like that if you are deficient in vitamins, especially the B range. Make sure you keep up your intake.

Major remedies to consider are:

Ignatia and *Pulsatilla* where there is mild depression with outbursts of weeping, soon after and probably in reaction to the birth.

If a more profoundly depressed state develops then consider *Sepia*, whose picture of aversion to loved ones and total loss of interest in anything at all is very like that of post-natal depression. It has even been given successfully to sheep who abandon their lambs. The mother will be weak, sad and tired. Everything will be too much for her, and she will be angry and aggressive to those around her as well as depressed and tearful.

If there is a very deep gloom, incessant talking and a very real desire to harm the baby, the remedy is *Cimicifuga*.

Do not delay in consulting a professional homoeopath if post-natal depression develops. It is easier to treat in its early stages.

A leaflet offering further information on the use of homoeopathy in pregnancy is available from the Society of Homoeopaths (see Appendix 2).

Chapter Eight

CHILDREN'S ILLNESSES

Children do not come into life flawless: they are born with predispositions to various types of personality and illness, and we cannot protect them against their genes. One of the functions of childhood is to develop a healthy and resilient immune system, which will provide a strong defence against ill-health for the rest of the person's life. One of the ways in which a child does this is by being exposed to and recovering from the various minor diseases of childhood.

The best way to protect children against disease and to give them a healthy start to life is to bring them up on a good healthy varied diet and to give them as much love, fresh air and fun as possible, and as few preservatives and drugs. This chapter will offer suggestions about the treatment of whatever children's ailments do come your way. Register with a homoeopathic practitioner so that you can discuss the finer points of your home treatment or join a local class teaching homoeopathic first aid. Look for details of these in your local library.

Children are easy to treat because most of their symptoms are very clear, undisguised as yet by politeness or the habit of putting up with or understating problems. The emphasis within homoeopathy on symptoms which represent small deviations from the norm of the patient's behaviour makes it particularly suitable for use by mothers, who are always first to sense when a child is not well, often before any physical symptoms appear, precisely because there are subtle changes not always obvious to others. It does not matter if the child cannot be precise about where it hurts or what they feel: you or the homoeopath will be able to see the important general picture well enough to prescribe: temperature, emotional state, change in colour are all excellent indications.

Most of the remedies useful in children's ailments are those mentioned over and over again in this book, and the principles for prescribing for them are the same. Children get over most of the afflictions of childhood without too much trouble, but it is often worrying to watch them do so, and using remedies can make their passage from illness back to health a lot smoother.

A small number of remedies can make a large difference to your capacity to deal with your children's health. If you can identify your child's basic remedy type, you will find that this remedy will help you in most of her illnesses, whatever the specific symptoms.

In the rest of this chapter I shall be discussing in detail eight remedies which cover most of the complaints arising in childhood. If you have these on hand you will be able to help your child a great deal and may never need any other remedies except in very specific circumstances, in the case of accidents and injuries, for instance. The remedies are *Aconite, Belladonna, Chamomilla, Hepar sulph, Merc sol, Pulsatilla, Silica* and *Sulphur.* These are all represented in the main *Materia Medica,* which should be consulted for fuller pictures. Here I have concentrated on the use of these remedies in illnesses commonly suffered by children. Naturally, if an adult finds herself in any of these states she can also use these remedies.

ACONITE

Aconite is a remedy for anything which comes on suddenly especially after exposure to cold dry weather or draughts or if the child has been frightened in any way. The child will be very hot, thirsty and restless, whatever the complaint. Give *Aconite* at the first sign that the child is coming down with something.

If there is a fever it will come on quickly with a severe chill followed by a high temperature. The child will be intensely thirsty for cold water. She will also be hot, red in the face (sometimes pale; sometimes one cheek will be red, one pale). She will kick off the bedclothes. Anxiety and fear may be marked and she will be extremely restless, worse in the evening, in a warm room and lying on the left side.

It is a remedy for the first stages of anything: coughs, colds, sore throats, croup, earache, measles. Give it quickly, especially in croup: if it is given in time, no other remedy will be needed. The cough is violent, dry, loud and barking. (Steam also helps relieve the symptoms quickly.) Use *Spongia* if the croupy cough does not respond to *Aconite* within a couple of hours, or if the child's breathing is still harsh, hard and barking. Give *Hepar sulph* in the third stage of croup, when there is infection.

In colds there will be frequent sneezing and a very painful burning throat. It is wonderful for the kind of earache that comes on after being in a cold wind: there will be an intense throbbing burning tearing pain and it will be worse for noise and warmth. It may also be of use in teething where the general symptoms apply.

In measles, give *Aconite* in the early stages before the rash comes out. There may be a catarrhal discharge from the nose and the eyes will be very sensitive to light.

BELLADONNA

Belladonna is often indicated in children, since it is suited to those who are normally robust and healthy but come down with a crash when ill. The child will have a red hot flushed face with no sweat (she sweats only on covered parts), she will be red hot and throbbing: you will be able to feel the heat coming from her skin.

Her eyes will be noticeably glittery with dilated pupils; she will be less restless than *Aconite*, more drowsy, she may be thirsty but not as much as *Aconite*. She will not be so fearful and anxious as *Aconite*, although in delirium she may see faces and horrible animals. She will be better for warmth and will not want to be uncovered, the opposite of *Aconite*.

There may be a lot of twitchy convulsive movements, especially in sleep. It can be used in convulsions that occur with teething. The child will be extremely sensitive to the light, will not be able to bear it.

It is an acute remedy for any inflammatory conditions marked by heat, redness, pain, tenderness, sensitivity and restlessness. So ears may be affected with acute earache, there may be sore throats, acute tonsillitis, scarlatina. The earache might tend to be in the right ear and be worse for sudden movement, touch or jarring, better for heat and stillness. *Belladonna* is indicated in the stage before there is any discharge. Wherever there is a rash it will be red, hot and dry: the unaffected skin will be pale. It may be indicated in German measles (rubella) with tender swollen glands in the neck.

There is an acute *Belladonna* rage and temper, when the child throws things and may kick and bite. This may be seen in fever or in children who become hyperactive for any reason. The reason is often sensitivity to sugar in any form, preservatives and colourings in food, especially tartrazine, the orange colouring, or to other chemicals. See how your child's behaviour changes if you take care to eliminate these things from her diet for a few days. If it does not change, allergy tests are available which may reveal a more idiosyncratic food sensitivity. (*Arsenicum alb*, *Chamomilla* and *Calcarea carbonica* should also be considered in the case of suspected food sensitivities).

CHAMOMILLA

The *Chamomilla* picture is very easy to recognize. The child is very irritable and cross; she will work herself up into a terrible temper, and nothing you do will be right even if you do what she asks. She will ask for a toy then throw it away when it's given to her. She won't want to be spoken to or even looked at. She is intensely restless and wants to move about all the time. Being carried is the only thing that will pacify her.

Whatever the complaint the pain will be terrible, unbearable. She will scream and scream and double up with pain. Sometimes she might even scream so much that she goes into convulsions.

The child is generally very hot whatever the complaint; she will have a hot head and burning feet. Her face will be flushed, often with one cheek pale, especially when teething or when she has a high temperature in fever. She will be generally very thirsty, especially for cold water.

The remedy is particularly indicated in colic and teething problems, especially where the two occur together. The child will be cross at night and have tender inflamed gums which may be relieved by cold applications. Toothache is improved by holding cold water in the mouth and can sometimes be brought on by warm things in the mouth. Colic is improved by hot applications. It usually comes on after anger or screaming: there is wind and greenish diarrhoea.

The remedy is also well indicated in earache; the child will not want to be touched and will be extremely irritable, feel the pain to be totally unbearable.

HEPAR SULPH

In *Hepar sulph*, probably the strongest characteristic is an oversensitivity which runs through the remedy both psychologically and physically. Children will be touchy, irritable, discontented and quarrelsome as well as being physically oversensitive to impressions, touch, surroundings, pain, cold.

Everything festers and suppurates. Everywhere feels sore and bruised as if there were a boil. Give it wherever there are pussy conditions, especially where the pus has come quickly, (*Silica* forms pus more slowly) in croup, abscesses, boils, whitlows, conjunctivitis, tonsillitis, ear infections.

Any infected part is extremely tender to touch and the slightest pressure causes a sharp pain, described as being like a splinter. When ill in bed, sufferers cannot bear the clothes to touch them or any touch; they are sensitive even to breaths of air, to the least draught, to putting even a hand outside the bedclothes.

Children may have a lot of catarrhal colds which start with an itchy throat and a lot of sneezing every time they go into a cold wind. The discharge is initially watery, later thick, yellow and offensive, smelling often like decomposed cheese.

All complaints are worse for cold. It is a great remedy in croup for sensitive children who have been exposed to cold air or dry cold winds and have come down with croup the following morning. The child is so sensitive to cold that the least exposure, even uncovering an arm or a foot, excites a spell of coughing.

Although adults have a constant thirst for sips of fluid, children may not be thirsty at all. They crave fatty and vinegary foods and get diarrhoea from eating juicy fruit and ice cream.

MERC SOL
Merc sol is a very useful remedy for children, since it covers some of the more vicious complaints to which they are subject. Ear, nose and throat problems predominate. These are the colds and earaches which have horrible stinking yellow or yellowy-green pussy burning discharges.

The glands in the throat and neck are inflamed and swollen in complaints such as tonsillitis and mumps. It often follows *Belladonna* in tonsillitis.

The child will salivate a lot, the saliva will drip out of the mouth onto the pillow at night. Mouth ulcers are common, as are toothache and abscesses in the teeth and mouth. There is often a metallic taste, a taste like silver paper.

Fevers are hectic with shivering restlessness and trembling and heavy sweating, especially at night: sweating does not relieve the fever.

It is a very pussy remedy: infections and wounds suppurate rapidly with burning and stinging. In chicken pox, the child will develop large pussy eruptions that become open sores. There may be repeated ear infections with offensive pussy discharges.

The child needing this remedy will be very hungry and thirsty, especially for cold milk and fizzy drinks, and will get an upset stomach from eating too many sweets.

The child may be very restless and impulsive, full of anxiety, will have fearful dreams. It is best suited to nervous children who talk very quickly and are inclined to stutter. They find it difficult to stay still, feel hurried inside. It is also indicated for mischievous, sometimes malicious, children who are always into things, restless, rushing from one thing to another.

PULSATILLA

A *Pulsatilla* child is affectionate and eager to please, also clingy, cannot let mother out of her sight. When ill she will become irritable and whingey, will not know what to do with herself, will refuse to be left alone and will need constant entertainment and reassurance.

If there is any fever, it will be low and slow without delirium; it may be accompanied by nausea and headache. The child's temperature will be erratic, one part of the body may be hot, another cold. She won't be thirsty even when complaining of a dry mouth.

Illnesses characteristically come on slowly and in a mild fashion and take a long time to clear up. There are often catarrhal complications, so, for example, after a cold the child may be deaf for a while or may have a stuffed-up nose long after the infection has passed. Colds tend to stay in the head: the nose will be blocked in warm rooms and at night, the cough will be dry and tickly at night. Both will be freer in the daytime and outdoors. It is indicated in hayfever.

Catarrhal ear problems are common, and glue ear is a strong feature. The child will be prone to earache with any condition and the earache will be worse from heat, evening and night, better in the open air and from cold applications. She will also readily get earache from exposure to cold.

Pulsatilla is usually chilly but dislikes the heat, and is better for fresh air and worse for warm stuffy rooms. In general, however, children are hotter than adults so do not rule out *Pulsatilla* if the child is not particularly chilly.

Everything is worse at dusk, night; cough is dryer at night, loose in day; everything is worse when lying down.

Gentle movements and pressure relieve: colic is better for gentle pressure on the abdomen, colds are better for gentle movement in the open air.

The digestion is weak: the child will be sick after parties because ice cream and cakes disagree with her, although she likes them. She may also be sick from the emotional excitement. She is particularly liable to digestive upsets if she gets cold or eats cold food after a hot spell.

She may sleep with her hands above her head.

SILICA

A child needing *Silica* is likely to appear quite thin (though need not be). She will have a tendency to lose weight. She may have difficulty assimilating food and her bones may not form well. She may have weak ankles, be slow learning to walk and slow teething; the fontanelles may close slowly.

These are the kind of children who don't thrive, who always have glandular problems or colds or earaches or abscesses. Everything seems to fester. They have septic cuts, whitlows, boils.

They feel the cold a lot, have icy cold hands and feet. They seem to lack stamina, look a bit delicate. They sweat profusely especially at night and on the back of the head and neck and they tend to have smelly sweaty feet (their socks rot).

They like cold food and drinks, hot drinks make them sweat, milk causes stomach upsets, babies cannot even digest the mother's milk. Such children can be fed on a specially prepared formula usually based on soya protein. They have a peculiar kind of constipation where the stool slips back just as it is about to emerge. They tend to get headaches which are better from heat and warmth and worse from cold or mental exertion.

The child may be restless and nervous, oversensitive to noise, especially small noises. She will be shy and lack confidence, dreading failure. However, in an effort to avoid failure she becomes very conscientious, always working hard to get things right. She likes to be sure of things before she speaks, but once she has made her mind up she will stick to it with great firmness, even to the point of obstinacy.

SULPHUR

Sulphur is a remedy for an enormous number of disease conditions. In children it will be found most useful in the numerous itchy skin conditions which afflict them, and it will be found particularly useful in clearing up long-standing complaints which drag on.

Like the adult, the child is active and restless, curious and open, a natural leader. The characteristic self-centredness is more acceptable in children and can be charming. If balked, however, the child may become irritable and whingey. They are messy and untidy, careless and chaotic, playing several games at once. They don't want to go to bed at night.

Common complaints among *Sulphur* children are headaches, which they get frequently, itchy skin, worse for washing, conjunctivitis, asthma and other chest infections.

They can be thin, hungry all the time and hyperactive, or tend to put weight on. They have a strong desire for sweets and spicy foods and a dislike of milk, sour food and eggs. They are thirsty, especially for ice-cold drinks.

They are warm-blooded, and intolerant of heat in any form. They also have a dislike of extreme cold. They are worse for stuffy atmospheres and getting overheated, and better for fresh air. Their feet get hot and they stick them out of bed at night.

First Aid

With the eight remedies detailed above, you should be able to deal with many children's complaints other than those caused by the frequent accidents to which they are prone. The following hints will help you choose remedies when they (or anyone else) need first aid for various minor injuries. You should always consult your health practitioner if any injury fails to respond quickly to remedies. Take the victim to hospital immediately in case of any serious injury, head injury, severe burns, suspected fractures, sprains or in any case where the pain seems disproportionate to the injury.

CREAMS AND LOTIONS

Calendula is the great homoeopathic 'antiseptic' to be used as a dressing for wounds, broken skin, abscesses and mouth ulcers. It is sometimes mixed with *Hypericum* tincture and called Hypercal.

The tincture can be diluted at a ratio of roughly ½ teaspoon to a quarter pint (about 150 ml) of water (boiled or sterile). The creams and ointments can be used freely when needed.

Nelson's Burn Ointment can be externally applied to burns, stings etc. *Arnica* ointment and tinctures may be applied to bruises and sore muscles if required, but never to an open wound.

Homoeopathy is unusual in using internal remedies to aid injuries: all the remedies referred to in the following section should be taken internally unless otherwise specified.

BITES AND STINGS
Apis (where there is swelling and burning as in a bee sting), *Cantharis* (where there is burning and stinging), *Hypericum* (very painful, especially from animals or horse flies), *Ledum* (irritating itching where scratching makes the itching worse), *Nat mur* (particularly in bee stings), *Staphysagria* (puncture wounds, sharp bites as of midges), *Urtica* (where itching predominates, as a nettle sting).

BLEEDING
Arnica (especially after a blow), *Ipecac, Belladonna, Phosphorus*: spontaneous nose bleeds.

BRUISES
Arnica (anywhere), *Hypericum* (parts rich with nerves: trapped or lacerated fingers, toes, fall on coccyx), *Ledum* (old stubborn bruising), *Ruta* (eyes, shins), *Symphytum* (shins, eyeball).

BURNS
In any burn there is an element of shock. Give *Aconite* or *Arnica* immediately; give *Calendula* tablets internally for minor (first degree) burns; *Cantharis* for blistering (second degree) burns; *Causticum* for third degree burns with severe skin loss – send for an ambulance and give the remedy while you are waiting; also for old burns. Give *Phosphorus* for electrical burns or shocks.

Externally apply soap, Aloe Vera gel (or the juice of the plant leaf) or Nelson's Burn Ointment to minor or other burns. Apply *Calendula* lotion to second degree burns when the blisters break.

CUTS AND SCRAPES
Calendula (torn jagged cuts especially), *Hypericum* (deep cuts affecting nerves); *Staphysagria* (clean cuts as from knives, especially to fingers).

Externally use *Calendula* tincture (diluted ½ teaspoon in a quarter pint/150 ml of water) or *Calendula* cream to keep wound clean.

EYE INJURY
Aconite or *Arnica* immediately (*Aconite* is called the *Arnica* of the eye); *Euphrasia* (conjunctivitis after injury); *Lachesis* (black eyes); *Symphytum* (blunt injury to eyeball).

Euphrasia tincture ½ teaspoon to a quarter pint/150 ml of sterile water roughly) can be used as an eyebath.

FRACTURES
Arnica, (especially soft tissues around fracture); *Bryonia* (where pain is much worse for movement); *Calc phos* (where bone nutrition is poor and is not healing); *Symphytum* (bone itself: use only after bone has been properly set).

HEAD INJURIES
Arnica (immediately); *Nat sulph* (head injury followed by headache or other ill effects). Go to hospital for a check even if everything seems all right.

HEAT EXHAUSTION/SUNSTROKE
Belladonna (better bending head backwards); *Glonoine* (worse bending head backwards).

PUNCTURE WOUNDS
Hypericum (to parts rich in nerves); *Ledum* (throbbing, pricking); *Staphysagria* (severe pain).

SHOCK
Aconite (distressed, anxious, fearful); *Arnica* (dull, stupid, will say is all right even though is clearly not); *Ignatia* (showing extremes of emotion, sighing, fainting, breathing very quickly).

STRAINS AND SPRAINS
Arnica (first); *Bryonia* (worse for movement); *Ledum* (especially ankles); *Rhus tox* (after the most acute symptoms have gone, worse after first movement, better with continued movement and heat); *Ruta* (use after initial tenderness and swelling decline a little).

Chapter Nine

THE MENOPAUSE

This is the time all women dread, but they need not. By the time we get to this stage we have usually forgotten what puberty was like, and so the sudden appearance of similar symptoms is a bit frightening. Hot flushes, mood swings, disturbances in the length of menstrual cycle, changes in the nature of the bleeding are all things which might happen over a period of as long as ten to fifteen years, while our hormones begin the process of adjustment for the later stages of life.

The myth of the menopause is stronger than the facts: for many women this period is relatively trouble-free, consisting mainly of mild hot flushes, increasingly irregular periods and a little dryness in the vagina, which may often be short-lived. Only about half of us have more than a few hot flushes, and most of us do not have them to a distressing level. Only a minority suffer from heavy bleeding, and it is usually associated with fibroids rather than hormonal change. Severe mood swings usually only affect those who have been prone to these at an earlier stage in life. Nevertheless, if you are one of the minority who do have difficulties with the menopause, you can have a very distressing time. Careful eating, attention to lifestyle and homoeopathy can help enormously to relieve this.

Many of the problems are emotional, to do with the mood

swings associated with unpredictable changes in the hormonal balance. Women begin to feel tired: so tired that they just can't get through what they used to get through. This is in itself distressing. Most women have very busy lives which depend on being 100 per cent fit. It takes a while to adjust to the fact that the tiredness is not just going to go away. Sleep can be disturbed, adding to the fatigue. For some people the menopause is like having pre-menstrual syndrome all the time, with that same emotional unpredictability.

There are a few remedies which are indicated generally for menopausal conditions because their characteristic symptoms embrace those which are also characteristic of the menopause: *Lachesis, Natrum mur* and *Sepia* are completely invaluable to the homoeopath at this time. It is at this time that many women may need these remedies, although they may never have done so before. A quick glance at their general pictures will make the reasons clear.

SEPIA

Sepia is very clearly a remedy associated with deficiencies of oestrogen and progesterone, lack of muscular tone and the congestion of blood in the veins. Difficulties with menstruation are a large part of its general picture: periods are usually delayed and there is either scanty flow or flooding. The *Sepia* exhaustion is marked just before and during the period, especially in the morning. Menopause is accompanied by hot flushes, fainting and anxiety; there may be bleeding between periods. The womb is often displaced because of a lack of tone in the muscles, usually dating from childbirth but not becoming a problem until the menopause. There is an intense bearing down sensation (as if everything were going to fall out through the vagina) along with pain in the lower back. This feeling is worse for standing or walking, so that the sufferer may feel that she has to sit down and cross her legs for support. There may be actual prolapse of womb and vagina. There is often leucorrhoea with a yellow or yellowish-green irritating, burning discharge. There may be dryness and itching of the vagina and pain on intercourse; there may also be erosion of the cervix. All this only adds further to the general loss of interest in sex characteristic of *Sepia*, especially where intercourse is involved.

LACHESIS

Lachesis is an equally important menopausal remedy. Hot flushes, fainting, floodings, melancholy and weakness are strongly present in its picture. In addition there may be cramps in the womb and profuse sweats. There are violent left-sided congestive headaches and left-sided ovarian pain (extending to the right) may be present.

A woman who needs *Lachesis* is characteristically worse after sleep and worse if the flow is delayed or suppressed. This makes the menopause a very difficult time for her: as the periods cease, so her mood becomes more and more difficult to manage. It is now that her tendency to suspiciousness, jealousy and rage might be at its most distressing. However, there will be no falling-off of interest in sex (unlike *Sepia*). It is also a remedy for older women who have never really got over the menopause, have never been well since then.

NATRUM MUR

Natrum muriaticum presents a completely different picture of menopausal symptoms, but one which is nevertheless common. Here the woman becomes more and more introverted, more and more the prisoner of her unexpressed feelings. Periods may become scanty and slight rather than more frequent with flooding, she feels full of tension all the time as if the period were about to start; she wants to be by herself to brood. She is extremely cross, resentful and irritable.

In this remedy too there will be a tendency to prolapse and dryness of the vagina, and naturally the woman will not be keen on sexual intercourse because it is uncomfortable; however, she will not have the same hostility to it as *Sepia*.

Any remedy may be used for complaints associated with the menopause, if the general symptoms agree of course, but these three are particularly likely to be indicated.

Hot Flushes

These may well respond to one of the following on a short term basis:

Belladonna where the face will be very red and hot, even throbbing. The woman will be restless, agitated and probably have palpitations as well.

Lachesis will have sweating with flushing and will often have violent headaches with it.

Pulsatilla may be indicated for milder hot flushes, probably brought on by being in a hot place. The rest of the body may be chilly and the woman may generally be tearful.

Sulphur where shivering precedes the hot flushes and there is a faint sensation at the same time.

Heavy Bleeding

The most frightening physical symptom of the menopause is undoubtedly that of heavy bleeding, even flooding or haemorrhaging. Heavy bleeding is often caused by fibroids, little lumps of muscle cells, in the womb. These are harmless in themselves, though, as with all 'new growths' there is an outside chance that they could become malignant. The real danger is that they might cause serious haemorrhaging, or miscarriage in younger women. They are often symptomless and usually shrink of their own accord after the menopause; if they cause a lot of trouble they may be modified, or even removed, by surgery. Heavy (and painful) bleeding may also be caused by endometriosis, excessive growth of the lining of the womb.

There are many remedies which can be used to balance the system to reduce the general tendency to heavy bleeding: remedies such as *China, Lachesis, Phosphorus* and *Sepia*, where haemorrhage is a strong characteristic. In *China* and *Phosphorus* debility from loss of blood, fatigue and exhaustion would be marked. *Lachesis* and *Sepia* would struggle to continue their strenuous lifestyles and become depressed and bad tempered as a result. *Lachesis* would characteristically feel better in herself once the flow was established, despite the heaviness. *Sepia* would show the characteristic bearing down, sagging sensation. *Kali carb* should be thought of where there is persistent heavy bleeding despite surgical or other intervention. *Natrum mur* may also have very heavy early periods (though they can also be scanty and delayed) at this time and will be likely to suffer from anaemia.

In an emergency heavy bleeding may be controlled in its acute phase with one of the following:

Belladonna, where the blood is bright red and hot with clots; there will be general congestion, throbbing and restlessness.

China, where the period is early and very heavy, the blood will be black and clotted and its loss will be accompanied by exhaustion and vertigo.

Ipecac, where there will be bright red blood accompanied by weakness, nausea and vomiting.

In cases of such heavy bleeding you may need to take the indicated remedy every half hour or so.

Vaginal Dryness

After the menopause is over, the chief problems may be osteoporosis and a general tendency for the body fluids to diminish, resulting in some dryness of the eyes, skin and vagina. Before the menopause we are protected against these things by a high level of oestrogen. Oestrogen production declines naturally after the menopause (since it is not needed so much) and because of this there is a tendency for the orthodox medical profession to advocate the use of Hormone Replacement Therapy (HRT). Although there is plenty of anecdotal evidence about the benefits of HRT, there are many unanswered questions about the ongoing and long-term effects of this treatment and it seems wisest to avoid it unless absolutely necessary. At the moment it seems possible that, while HRT can definitely stop hot flushes, night sweats and vaginal dryness as well as delaying the onset of osteoporosis, it can also increase the risk of gall bladder disease, breast and endometrial cancer. Also, there comes a point when you need to stop the HRT and face the facts of the ageing process. Unless the symptoms of menopause are really severe and cannot be dealt with in other ways, it seems wise to cope with this change of state while you are still young.

Dryness of the vagina can be helped by homoeopathic remedies and food supplements. Vitamin E has proved helpful in many cases. Ginseng may also be temporarily helpful since it appears to raise the levels of oestrogen in the body. If the dryness makes sexual activity uncomfortable, lubricants such as KY Jelly make a big difference. *Calendula* cream may also be used for this purpose.

Remedies such as *Bryonia, Lycopodium, Natrum muriaticum, Sepia* and *Staphysagria* have an obvious relationship to the drying-out process and, where indicated, may correct the imbalance.

Bryonia is the best-indicated remedy, as it generally affects the fluid in all the mucous membranes: the symptoms of dryness might be accompanied by weakness in the chest and a tendency to constipation. In the case of *Lycopodium*, the problem is more likely to be dryness of the external skin accompanied by flatulence and indigestion. *Natrum mur*'s dryness will be mucosal like that of *Bryonia*, accompanied by the classic symptoms of fluid retention and emotional reserve. *Sepia*'s dryness will be accompanied by soreness and loss of interest in sexual intercourse. *Staphysagria*'s dryness will be likely to be made more painful by sexual intercourse.

Osteoporosis

The thought of developing osteoporosis scares many women into accepting HRT, which is guaranteed to prevent it. Osteoporosis is thinning of the bone caused by a loss of calcium. In both men and women the bones cease to replace themselves with age; however, this process only leads to something as definite as osteoporosis in 1 in 4 women. Where it does develop, it seems to be connected with the loss of oestrogen that occurs with and after the menopause; while oestrogen and progesterone therapy can slow down the rate of bone loss after the menopause, bone that has already been lost cannot be replaced. Furthermore, bone loss will be delayed only as long as the treatment lasts.

There are many ways of avoiding the development of osteoporosis other than the use of HRT. The most efficient and the one which leads to the best general overall health is, of course, to adopt a healthy lifestyle, including regular exercise and a healthy diet rich in calcium *well before* the menopause. Recommended amounts of calcium daily for pre-menopausal women are 1000mg and for post-menopausal women 1500mg. It is difficult to get this amount from the diet, since calcium is most readily available in dairy products which we are all busy avoiding because of their fat content! Other high calcium foods include oily fish such as sardines and salmon, almonds, tofu (and other soya products) and broccoli. You may want to take calcium supplements to make sure you get the right amount of calcium. Calcium supplements should always be taken in conjunction with magnesium.

However, this process is not as straightforward as it seems because there are many factors (not yet completely understood) which interfere with the absorption of calcium. The best course of action is probably to make sure that you get plenty of exercise and enough calcium from diet and supplements, and also have homoeopathic constitutional treatment to give your system the best chance to absorb the calcium. There are also remedies which have a specific action on the bone: *Calc carb, Calc fluor, Calc phos, Silica* and *Symphytum,* for instance; however, as always, the treatment which is likely to be successful is that which takes the whole person into account.

It cannot be stressed too strongly that many of the problems loosely referred to as women's problems are extremely amenable to homoeopathic treatment. Because most of these are based in the constitution and are not acute or minor problems amenable to first aid treatment, you should consult a homoeopathic practitioner about them. The purpose of this section has been to communicate a sense of the possibilities inherent in homoeopathy rather than to suggest that these often deeply-entrenched patterns of health can be removed by one remedy. If you suffer from such conditions as vaginal warts, cervical erosion, endometriosis, Pelvic Inflammatory Disease, ovulation problems, infertility, ovarian cysts or fibroids there is strong possibility that an experienced homoeopath will be able to help you with these.

Chapter Ten

AGEING

We live in a very youth-oriented culture at the moment. A woman as she becomes older may not feel, as would be appropriate, that she has become more centred, wiser and more respected, but rather that she is no longer desirable, and no longer has her looks. Fortunately, older people seem to be fighting back, with movements like the Grey Panthers and the University of the Third Age, so perhaps we do not have to go directly to the scrap heap as soon as we have passed the menopause. Nevertheless it is inevitable as we get older that a certain amount of wear and tear becomes apparent. There are ways of making the process, if not slower, at least more gracious, and of keeping some control over our own slow physical decline.

Circulation

As we get older, the blood doesn't seem to reach out to the edges of our body in quite the same way it once did. We develop all sorts of niggly problems to do with circulation: feet and hands get colder, chilblains may occur, varicose veins get more troublesome and may even ulcerate. The ankles and the bottom of the legs begin to look puffy and we start to worry in an undefined way about heart attacks and strokes. The best protection against all these is gentle exercise, good diet and doing what you want to be doing as far as possible.

I am not proposing that you treat serious circulatory problems with first aid remedies. However, we can follow the same principle as we have been following throughout the book. If you treat either yourself or someone else while the problem is still at a minor level, then you are contributing towards halting the advance to a more serious level. Even when the problem is serious you can sometimes help. You could, for instance, treat with first aid remedies the immediate effects of a stroke, while waiting for other help: this could make a considerable difference to the future quality of life of the victim.

If you have any sort of heart problems, you should see a practitioner who will be able to help you with such common and chronic conditions as angina, high blood pressure, heart disease and phlebitis.

Palpitations and Fainting

Palpitation is a sensation that the heart is beating irregularly or faster or harder than it should. It can be a symptom of heart disease, but in nine out of ten cases it is caused merely by a disturbance in the nervous control of the heart and often associated with indigestion. The heart and stomach are controlled by the same nerve, so any injury to one is often felt sympathetically by the other.

Aconite will help, especially where fear is the cause.

Ignatia is useful where any kind of emotional upset is involved, or where the palpitations come on after eating.

Nux vomica may be useful where eating unusual food seems to be the cause.

Lachesis may be useful in the post-menopausal period when symptoms reminiscent of the menopausal stage recur randomly, and you may suffer from feelings of fainting, constricted feeling in the chest and anxiety with palpitations.

Chilblains

These may not be serious but they can be very painful. *Pulsatilla*, with its picture of permanently disordered circulation, is the remedy most likely to help. *Agaricus* is a specific remedy for the sort of burning prickling pains associated with chilblains. *Arsenicum* has the familiar symptoms of burning and itching, worse for cold.

Collapse

The *Carbo veg* picture includes a slowing down of the circulation, exhaustion, weakness, prostration and a tendency to collapse and faint. It is known as the 'corpse reviver'. It should be given in any case of collapse, whatever the cause, while waiting for other help. Some causes might be food poisoning, carbon monoxide poisoning, hypothermia, weakness after an operation. The body and breath will be cold, face and lips blue. Put the victim into the first aid 'rescue position' before giving the remedy and crush the tablet to a powder before placing in the mouth.

Cramp

This is another very painful complaint which is often neglected because it appears to be minor. *Pulsatilla* is the chief remedy to be considered here. *Arsenicum*, *Arnica*, *Carbo veg*, *Causticum* and *China* may all also be helpful, depending on what other symptoms are present.

Often cramp is caused by a lack of calcium and magnesium, and supplements will help.

Phlebitis

This is inflammation of one of the superficial veins in the leg, caused by the formation of blood clots. It is not in itself serious but can lead to septicaemia (if there is infection) or embolism (fragmenting of blood clots which can then travel round the body to larger veins).

The following homoeopathic remedies may ease the symptoms while waiting for expert treatment.

Arnica, especially if the condition has been caused by an injury.

Hamamelis, where there is bruising and soreness.

Atherosclerosis/Arteriosclerosis

Both these terms refer to the hardening and narrowing of the arteries. In atherosclerosis the main cause is the deposit of fatty tissue (atheroma) in the arteries; in arteriosclerosis the narrowing is caused by loss of elasticity in the vessels.

Degenerative changes to the arteries begin in middle age, if not before. The walls of the blood vessels progressively lose elasticity and therefore don't dilate as they should to allow the free passage of the blood to brain and heart.

The effects of this chronic condition can vary considerably, from occasional dizziness to a heart attack or a stroke. As usual the best approach is prevention, or delay, by the adoption of a diet low in animal fats and alcohol and high in fibre, vegetables and fruit. If acute symptoms occur it may be useful to use *Arnica*, a great emergency remedy for stroke.

Confusion

This is one of the most distressing features of ageing. Leaving aside any emotional causes, it is usually a sign that the blood supply to the brain is being interrupted in some way. If this has been the result of a fall or injury then give *Arnica*. If it is as a result of hypothermia (chronic loss of body temperature) then give *Carbo veg*.

Sudden confusion may have more serious causes, so call the doctor or your health practitioner if you are in any doubt.

Dizziness/Vertigo

In old people this is most likely to be due to hardening of arteries leading to impairment of the balancing mechanisms.

Arnica, *Bryonia*, *Causticum*, and *Conium* may all be helpful.

Varicose Veins

Hamamelis and *Pulsatilla* are both useful in the case of chronic varicose veins. They relieve the pain and swelling. It is also a good idea to rest with the legs elevated above the heart. If the veins itch, a little witch hazel lotion (from chemists) may relieve them.

If the veins are ulcerated and broken then take *Calendula* tablets internally and apply *Calendula* ointment. If you are having the sores dressed by a nurse, she will usually be willing to try applying the *Calendula* instead of the orthodox ointment. This can bring about a remarkable improvement.

Carbo veg might also be indicated in the itching varicose veins of old age; *Lachesis* may be needed in severe cases where there is purple inflammation; *Belladonna* will do well where the inflammation is a brighter red.

Muscles and Joints

These are usually among the first parts to give problems. For some, of course, trouble with muscles and joints will have started well before this time. Rheumatoid arthritis and similar rheumatic affections of the immune system tend to strike earlier in life. But for most women, pain and stiffness in the muscles and joints only become a chronic problem in the later years.

Arthritis and rheumatism are among the commonest diseases to affect the population of Western countries. In most cases the causes are unclear and the orthodox treatment ineffective. This is the condition of which doctors say, even more than usual: 'you'll have to live with it'. In fact, in many cases, you won't. Though the gradual degeneration of the bone associated with osteoarthritis may be inevitable once it has begun, the severe pain that sometimes goes with it is not, and the degeneration itself can be modified by careful diet and exercise. It has become clear that there are many causes of muscle and joint pain. While some conditions are intractable, most can be halted and relief from pain obtained by a variety of approaches, including diet, food supplements and homoeopathic remedies.

A great deal of muscle and joint pain seems to be caused by eating the wrong kind of food and accumulating toxins in the tissues. Sometimes stress prevents the body from dealing with food in the way it should. Sometimes food sensitivity or the rarer allergy is involved. Poor nutrition will affect the whole body, including the muscles and joints, and if the body cannot metabolize calcium properly too much will be deposited, distorting and thickening the joints, or too little, depleting the bones of this essential mineral. Some pain is due to poor lubrication: the fluid which surrounds all the joints needs to have certain minerals and proteins in it to be an efficient lubricator. If these are lacking or the cells are poisoned with toxins, lubrication will be inadequate.

So the first step to ridding yourself of muscle and joint pain is to adopt a good diet. The basic diet should consist of fresh, whole foods, as many as possible raw. Starches and sugar should be at an absolute minimum. There are many books available suggesting a variety of different 'arthritis' diets, and you should experiment until you find the one that suits you. What suits one person in terms of diet won't be what suits another. Both the Hay diet and the Dong diet have helped many people: see Appendix 1 for books containing these.

In the face of such an obviously constitutional state, a homoeopathic practitioner should be consulted for the best results. However, there are a number of remedies which may be used in acute manifestations of the more chronic condition: these may prevent too much damage occurring and give some relief from debilitating pain.

ARNICA

With its picture of generalized soreness and bruised sensations, this is a good all-purpose remedy for pain and is always to be used first in the case of any fall or injury. It prevents and relieves muscle aches, strains and fatigue from over-exertion. It is good in cases of rheumatism where the patient is sore all over, and so tender to touch as to wish to avoid being approached. Joints are inflamed, shining, red and hard; the bed feels too hard. It is also useful in gout.

BRYONIA

Symptoms include pain with slight redness, heat and swelling. Pains are likely to have been brought on by cold east winds and tend to be stitching and predominantly right-sided. *Bryonia* is worse for movement, better for rest and pressure, and even tight bandaging; is also often relieved by cold applications.

RHUS TOX

Symptoms include pain usually with slight redness, heat and swelling, brought on by or worse in damp weather. The pains are tearing and tend to move round the body from joint to joint, worse at rest, better for heat and better for movement, though the first movement in the morning or after prolonged rest is the most painful. There is often restlessness, especially in bed at night. Better for warm dry applications: hot water bottle in the small of the back, for instance.

RUTA

This is similar to *Rhus tox* but more applicable to tendons and ligaments than to muscles. It is well-indicated in injury, strains and sprains of ligaments around the joints, and of the attachments of muscles and tendons, especially at the wrists and ankles. It is also indicated in injuries to the periosteum (bone covering beneath the skin). There is a sensation of weariness and of being bruised all over. The pain is worse for cold and wet and is helped by movement.

CAUSTICUM

This is particularly associated with the muscle and joint complaints of age. There is weakness and progressive loss of muscular strength. The joints are very stiff and often deformed, and it is suited to chronic rheumatic conditions. A notable feature is that it is worse in cold dry weather and better for damp wet weather. It is often accompanied by paralytic sensations, such as writer's cramp, and it can have tearing pains in the limbs. It is useful in complaints affecting only one part, for example the joints of the jaw or neck or a facial paralysis.

NUX VOMICA

Nux vomica is a great rheumatic remedy, very similar to *Causticum*. It is chilly and the sufferer is apt to get lumbago after getting cold. There is acute spasmodic pain, worse for motion, for draughts, for dry cold weather, better for warmth, rainy weather. Clearly, it is also likely to be useful where the muscle and joint pain is due to a buildup of toxins in the system over a lifetime.

Backache

All these remedies may be useful in lumbago or low backache, where the symptoms agree. Backache often needs physical treatment by osteopathy, massage, physiotherapy or chiropractic to allow the remedies space to do their best. *Hypericum* is a useful remedy to have for those painful occasions when your feet disappear from under you in the street or on the stairs, and you land on your tailbone. After such a jar to the body there is often substantial pain. *Symphytum* will be found invaluable in speeding up the knitting of bone and the healing after any fractures. It's useful if bone pains continue after the injury has apparently healed.

Incontinence

This is not an inevitable part of ageing, but involuntary loss of urine can be quite common. In women the main reason is 'stress incontinence' (momentary loss of bladder control when laughing, sneezing, coughing) caused by weakness of pelvic floor muscles. It usually starts in middle age but of course continues into old age if it is not sorted out. Incontinence can also be caused by infection or by constipation where the over-full bowel exerts pressure on the bladder.

Well-indicated remedies are *Gelsemium* in which all the muscles are weak, *Causticum* with its strong toning action on the bladder muscles, *Pulsatilla* where incontinence is worse for laughing, sneezing, lying on the back. *Petroselinum* is probably the best all-purpose assistance in night-time incontinence.

Pelvic floor exercises will be useful.

Faecal incontinence is less common than urinal incontinence but can be very distressing, and can also often prevent an elderly person from getting the kind of residential care they might need. Think first of *Gelsemium, Sepia,* and *Sulphur.*

PART TWO

Materia medica

Abbreviated Name	Remedy
Aconite	Aconitum napellus
Apis	Apis mellifica
Arg nit	Argentum nitricum
Arnica	Arnica montana
Arsenicum	Arsenicum album
Bella	Belladonna
Bryonia	Bryonia alba
Calc carb	Calcarea carbonica
Caust	Causticum
Cham	Chamomilla
China	China
Cimi	Cimicifuga (Actea racemosa)
Gelsemium	Gelsemium sempervirens
Hepar sulph	Hepar sulphuris calcareum
Ignatia	Ignatia amara
Ipecac	Ipecacuanha
Kali carb	Kali carbonicum
Lach	Lachesis
Lyc	Lycopodium clavatum
Merc sol	Mercurius solubilis
Natrum mur	Natrum muriaticum
Nux vom	Nux vomica
Phos	Phosphorus
Phytolacca	Phytolacca decandra
Pulsatilla	Pulsatilla nigricans
Rhus tox	Rhus toxicodendron
Sepia	Sepia
Silica	Silica
Staph	Staphysagria
Sulph	Sulphur

Cantaris?

Materia Medica

Aconitum napellus
(Aconite, monk's hood, wolf's bane)

A person who needs *Aconite* may suffer from severe anxiety and panic attacks. She may have a great fear of death (even a strong sense that it will take place at a specific time); she will be terrified of crowds, of open spaces, of going out, of the dark. These sudden panicky states are often accompanied by palpitations and flushing. Fear accompanies almost all complaints. It is a remedy for shock and for the effects of shock, even years after the event.

It is a remedy for the very earliest stages of complaints, the initial stages of inflammation and pain. In acute illnesses the patient will be terribly restless, will have a red dry hot flushed face (sometimes pale), burning skin (worse for warmth of bedclothes) and will be extremely thirsty for large quantities of cold water – everything else will taste bitter. She will be extremely sensitive to light, noise and touch.

Her circulation is very easily affected and there may be sudden flushing, raised blood pressure, swift alternation of heat and chill in fever, hot flushes in the menopause; palpitations are common.

It has been described as being like a big storm that soon blows over. The symptoms can disappear as quickly as they come.

Better: open air, rest, warm sweat (in acute cases).

Worse: cold dry wind, getting chilled, night especially midnight, fright, shock, noise, light.

Aconite symptoms come on **suddenly, violently** and **intensely** with **anxiety, fear** and **restlessness. Intense burning, tingling, shooting pains** are characteristic and **complaints** are often **brought on by getting chilled,** being **exposed to cold dry weather** or by **fright** or **shock.** There is a **red, dry, flushed face** and **burning** skin.

Where the general symptoms agree it should be considered in acute anxiety, colds (first stages), convulsions, coughs (dry), croup, earache, fevers, headaches, high blood pressure, hot flushes, labour pain, measles, neuralgia, palpitations, panic attacks, period pain, shock, sore throats, stroke, sun (heat) stroke, teething.

Apis mellifica (Honey bee)

The action of *Apis* is like the effects of a bee sting. There is sudden and dramatic swelling and inflammation with rosy redness, burning stinging pains, itching and a lot of general discomfort. The swellings feel tense and stiff and look puffy and watery. The pains are sudden and sharp and make the victim cry out; they may wander around the body. All symptoms are better for cold and much worse for heat.

In severe cases of bee stings the swelling can spread to any of the mucous membranes, so there may be watery swelling around the eyes, eyelids, mouth, face, joints or limbs or even swelling in the throat which makes breathing difficult. There may be urticaria-like eruptions on the skin with intolerable itching and burning. It is often indicated in allergic reactions which cause swelling in the mucous membranes or itchy swelling on the skin.

It has a high fever where the patient is hot, tearful, irritable, sleepy and delirious. The skin is hot and dry and sweaty by turn.

The body is generally sore and sensitive, worse for touch. Eyes and lips may be highly inflamed, swollen. There is a drowsy stupefied state which may be seen before the eruption comes out in measles. It is also highly indicated in meningitis.

It is a major remedy in cystitis, having frequent urging but inability to pass more than very small amounts of water at a time. There is sharp burning and stinging pain. It is also well indicated in rheumatic pain of a burning and stinging nature with red shiny swellings, especially in knees and toes.

The itching and burning manifests psychologically and emotionally in restlessness, unpredictability, irritability, fearfulness and suspiciousness, sometimes amounting to mania. There is also a depressed, apathetic state with a fear of being alone or of death. Jealousy is a strong characteristic of this remedy. It may be needed after a fright, rage, vexation or hearing bad news.

The sufferer tends to be warm-blooded and will be notably thirstless, even in fever. Kidney problems may develop. Symptoms are either right-sided or start on the right and move or spread to the left.

Better: cold in any form, fresh air, cold bathing, uncovering; change of position, walking about.

Worse: heat in any form, warm stuffy rooms, hot drinks, hot compresses, sleep, touch, pressure, late afternoon (4 p.m.), lying down.

Apis is characterized by **sudden inflammation** and **watery swelling** with **burning stinging pains** which make the patient **shriek**. The inflammation is **rosy red** and much **worse for heat, better for cold**. The patient is **thirstless** and **restless**. There is enormous **sensitivity** to **touch**.

Where the general symptoms agree it might be indicated in allergies, asthma, bites and stings, conjunctivitis, cystitis, fever, hay fever, mastitis, meningitis, mumps, ovaritis, PMS, prickly heat, sore throats, styes, synovitis, urticaria.

Argentum nitricum (Silver nitrate)

Time passes too slowly for anyone who needs this remedy: the sufferers always want to hurry things up. They feel driven and tormented by anxious and impulsive thoughts: they want to jump from windows and high places and into water, although they are afraid of heights, of tall buildings, of open spaces. They are extremely nervous of people and crowds.

Anticipatory anxiety is very strong in the remedy. Sufferers tremble with nervous excitement and get diarrhoea before exams or performance. They worry about being late for trains or appointments, about being alone, about their health. They are always expecting something unpleasant to happen, always wondering, 'What if . . .?'

They are terrified of failure and of criticism, chronically doubting their ability to succeed at anything. When they are under prolonged stress they may become mentally confused and forget things easily; they will be inclined to palpitations and trembling. This state might be chronic and constitutional or it might have been brought on temporarily by overwork, stress, studying for exams. It can also be brought on by some degenerative diseases.

There is extreme tiredness; exhaustion and trembling often come on after overwork and there can be difficulties with coordination, both mentally and physically.

Characteristically the sufferer is very warm-blooded, completely unable to bear heat of any kind, and suffers agonies in warm stuffy rooms. She is much better for fresh air and cold. Hot stuffy atmospheres make her feel claustrophobic.

The woman who needs *Arg nit* often has a feeling that parts of her are too big, for instance her head may feel as if it is squeezed in a vice or she may have a feeling that there is an iron band round her chest or waist. She frequently describes a sensation as if a splinter were stuck somewhere, in the throat, vagina or stomach for example. Ulceration is strong in the remedy.

The person who needs this remedy has a sweet tooth and craves sugar and sweets, but these cause sickness and diarrhoea. Flatulence and wind is marked. She gets diarrhoea with flatulence from nervousness or too many sweets. She also desires salty things and cold drinks and cold food.

The remedy tends to have left-sided complaints.

Better: cool fresh air, pressure on the affected part (especially headaches).

Worse: emotion, anxiety, in closed places, warmth, heat, stuffy rooms, eating sweets, sugar, cold food, intellectual work, emotional stress.

The woman who needs this remedy is **nervous, impulsive, restless, excitable** and **hurried,** suffering from enormous **anticipatory anxiety** which is often associated with **flatulence** and **diarrhoea. Tremulousness, weakness** and **paralysis** are also characteristic. The patient **feels** the **heat** excessively, **craves fresh air** and experiences **splinter-like** pains and sensations. **Craves sugar** and **sweets.**

It may be indicated in agoraphobia, anxiety, claustrophobia, conjunctivitis, diarrhoea, gastric pains, headaches, problems with menopause or menstruation, period pain, stomach ulcers.

Arnica montana (Leopard's bane)

Arnica has widespread sensations of bruising, soreness, stiffness and swelling. There is easy bleeding and bruising. Exhaustion and weariness are a strong feature, extreme tiredness with a bruised sore feeling. It is the remedy to think of immediately after any injury or accident. It prevents or brings down the bruising and swelling and helps alleviate the shock reaction. The sufferer feels as if she has been beaten up.

Think of it in threatened miscarriage, after delivery of a baby, after operations, hard physical exertion, concussion or where muscles are sore from unaccustomed exercise, in sore swollen joints, tennis elbow, etc. It is a major remedy for sprains, strains or breaks with pain, inflammation and swelling, especially in the first stage after the injury. You can think of it also if anyone feels bruised and sore without having been involved in an accident. It is useful for the effects of tiredness, overwork; after a sleepless night, for jet lag. When she is so tired the sufferer is characteristically very sensitive to heat, cold, touch of any sort: even the bed feels hard.

The emotional state associated with *Arnica* is something like the effect of concussion. The sufferer will deny being ill and will say she is well; she may be hopeless and indifferent and in a sort of stupor; may forget words while speaking and will not want to be touched or even approached. She wants to be left alone. Following an actual injury she may be fearful, forgetful, find concentration difficult. She may be despairing and morose. There is also a more actively bad-tempered state where the person is anxious, apprehensive about the future, quarrelsome, opinionated and obstinate.

It is an important remedy for bleeding, not only from external wounds but internally: bruises easily. Causes and cures small boils, broken small veins, bleeding, haemorrhage and septic states.

Better: first movement, worse as movement continues. Better rest and lying down with head lower than feet.

Worse: heat, exposure to hot sun, rest, jarring, lying on injured part, the slightest touch, cold, damp, movement, exertion, injuries, falls.

Arnica is **bruised, sore, stiff** and **swollen**. She **fears being touched**. It is the first remedy to use in case of **accidents and injuries**.

It may be indicated in abscesses that do not mature, accidents, boils, childbirth and its after-effects, gout, haemorrhages in the eye or under the skin, headaches, head injuries, muscle and joint pain, nosebleeds, shock, sprains, stings, stroke, after surgery, whooping cough.

Do not use it after tooth extraction as the speed with which this remedy stops internal bleeding may cause 'dry socket'.

Arsenicum album (White trioxide of arsenic)

Anxiety and restlessness are the fundamental characteristics of this remedy. The restlessness is both physical and psychological: the sufferer cannot sit still, tosses and turns, must be moving from place to place, or from one position to another. All pains and conditions are better for movement. She is always on the go, always ordering and tidying her environment.

Emotionally too she is restless: her anxiety takes many forms, shifting from one focus to another: health, death, the future, being alone, money. Anxiety about health is strongest: the sufferer fears germs and disease, notices the smallest deviations from perfect health, looks after her own and her family's health very well, taking up exercise and paying careful attention to diet. She is serious and earnest and perhaps a little timid.

In health this overactive, restless type of person may find it difficult to relax, but is nevertheless a competent and happy human being. As long as this temperament is able to express itself freely its owner can function in a practical and efficient way in the world, with a valuable and constructive orderliness. However, in a state of ill-health the natural fastidiousness may become a fanatical compulsive rigidity, a desperate attempt to keep the disorder of the external world at bay, to control an environment increasingly seen as hostile. The person may become obsessional, tidying and cleaning for the sake of it; a sensible attention to cleanliness and hygiene may turn into an obsessional fear of germs and dirt; a liking for accuracy and attention to detail become a dogmatic pedantry.

The sufferer can become critical and censorious, turning her angry feelings onto the outside world and blaming others who do nothing properly. In extreme cases a near paranoia may develop: she may come to fear that she has done wrong, offended people, become convinced that her friends hate her; she feels enormous guilt. The more she fears, the more she has to control her environment. She may become anorexic. She may become afraid of her own impulses, fearful of harming herself or others, she may develop a fear of knives.

All symptoms are worse at night, especially midnight and 3 a.m. She is afraid of the dark, afraid of dying, afraid of serious illness. She has anxious dreams and nightmares: of the dead, of danger, of pursuit. She is restless during sleep. She feels much better if she is in company, better if she is occupied.

There is also a very prostrated side to the remedy. This can emerge in feverish illnesses when the patient quickly becomes too weak to move about. The prostration seems out of all proportion to the condition. She is better then for rest but remains restless even in exhaustion, not least because the exhaustion makes her anxious. In more chronic states the desperate anxiety and driven mode of life tires her so much that she comes to a sort of paralysed standstill. She can also tire herself out through lack of sleep caused by anxiety and an overactive mind. She wakes in the early morning and worries about the coming day.

Physically *Arsenicum* is very chilly, extremely sensitive to cold. She has cold hands and feet. She is much better for warmth and heat except that her headache is better for fresh air.

There may be burning pains anywhere in the body but especially in the throat, eyes or stomach. The burning pains are better for heat, like other *Arsenicum* symptoms. The characteristic thin watery discharges also burn: the nose runs and burns in colds, diarrhoea burns the skin.

It is a major remedy for digestive problems: sickness and

diarrhoea are common in response to both food and anxiety. The sufferer tends to vomit easily and often; sometimes she cannot bear the sight, smell or thought of food. It is one of the most important remedies to think of in food-poisoning, especially if tinned meat or shellfish is suspected (*Carbo veg* is another important remedy here). There can be indigestion with burning pains, heartburn which is relieved by hot drinks. Warm food and drinks are favoured. She is thirsty but likes frequent small sips of cold water. It is obviously likely to be an important remedy in stomach ulcers and in ulcerative colitis, this type of person being the ulcer-prone personality.

The anxiety and oversensitivity to the environment is also reflected in the chest: there are difficulties with breathing and asthmatic complaints related both to anxiety and allergic reactions: hay fever, asthma. There is a characteristic dry hacking cough worse at night.

Better: for heat and warmth, (except headaches), company, brisk movement, walking about, open air, lying down, hot drinks.

Worse: cold air or applications, midnight till 3 a.m., cold ices, foods, cold and damp, vegetables, watery fruits, bad meat, change of temperature, exertion, wet weather, symptoms on right side.

The person who needs *Arsenicum* is extremely **anxious** and **restless**. She cannot be still either emotionally or physically. She is a **perfectionist, critical** and demanding. Physically she is very **chilly, better** for **warmth**, prone to **vomiting** and **diarrhoea, worse midnight** and till 3 a.m. **Burning pains** which are **better for heat** are characteristic. She can be extremely **weak** and **exhausted, prostrated** out of all proportion to the illness.

If the general symptoms agree this remedy might be considered in anorexia, anxiety, asthma, burns, chilblains, colds, cystitis, depression, diarrhoea and vomiting, digestive complaints, food poisoning, hay fever, high blood pressure, PMS, sleeplessness, stomach ulcers, ulcerative colitis, vaginitis.

Belladonna
(Atropa belladonna, deadly nightshade)

Sudden intense congestions and flushing are characteristic of this remedy: the skin (mainly the head and face) and mucous membranes are a bright shiny red. There is intense burning and stinging in the inflamed parts: ears, throat and stomach all burn and swell rapidly; the patient is very sensitive to touch and everything feels as if it were about to burst open. Pains are intense, pulsing and throbbing or spasmodic and cramp-like: they begin and end suddenly. Blood vessels throb and pulse, as do local inflammations.

The remedy is often indicated immediately after *Aconite* has stopped working or where the inflammation is more localized to the head and throat area. (*Aconite* inflammation is more general and the patient is thirstier.)

The patient is extremely physically sensitive and easily affected by jarring, touch, movement; she cannot lie on the painful side. Though not particularly responsive to outside temperatures, she will be sensitive to draughts, especially on the head. She is usually thirstless – she may be thirsty, but thirst is not characteristic of *Belladonna* as it is of *Aconite*. She may crave lemons or lemonade when thirsty. When ill she wants to be warmly wrapped. Complaints tend to be right-sided.

The patient is less fearful than is an *Aconite* patient and a child is more inclined to have tantrums and hit out and bite in rage. The very disturbed emotional state associated with *Belladonna* is most commonly seen in fevers but may also be seen in severe forms of mental illness. There is delirium and mania, the sufferer is very restless and agitated, talks very quickly, sees monsters, lives in her own world.

A person needing *Belladonna* will tend to have congested headaches with throbbing pains worse for any movement;

throbbing earaches, red hot dry itchy burning skin rashes. She will be inclined to catch colds and may develop a raw, red sore throat worse on the right side and worse swallowing liquids with a violent, dry, barking cough. In haemorrhages the blood is bright red and clotted; there are violent, cramp-like period pains. It is well-indicated in the menopause and for any person with high blood pressure, even in stroke. It is useful in urinary tract inflammation and skin infections.

Better: pressure, rest, warmth, light warm wraps.

Worse: motion, jarring, touch, pressure, cold, light, noise, 3 p.m., night, getting head wet, draughts to head, lying on the painful side, sun (sunstroke), heat, lying down.

Belladonna symptoms come on **suddenly, violently** and **intensely** and go as quickly. The remedy picture is characterized by **intense heat, redness, throbbing** and **swelling. Pains** are **burning.** There is **restlessness** and **extreme sensitivity to light, noise, touch.** Complaints tend to be **right-sided** and are often accompanied by **twitching, convulsive movements.**

It might be considered in abscesses, heavy bleeding, breast soreness, colds, convulsions, earache, fever, headache, high blood pressure, hot flushes, infectious diseases of children, inflammatory conditions, menopause, migraine, ovarian pain, piles, rheumatism, sinusitis, sore throat, sunstroke, tonsillitis, vertigo.

Bryonia alba
(White bryony or Wild hop)

The person who needs *Bryonia* will be extremely irritable, especially if anyone tries to disturb or move her at all. The sufferer wants to be alone when ill, resents being ill and wants to get back to work. She is touchy, morose, disgruntled and does not want to be talked to or interfered with in any way. She worries about money, security and business, is discontented and does not really know what she wants. Children don't want to be carried or moved about: they ask for things and then reject what's offered. They are capricious.

Irritability is also characteristic of the physical symptoms. Any movement at all makes the symptoms worse: you'll see people with a *Bryonia* headache holding their heads or tying them up in a scarf, people with a bad chest holding their ribs when they cough and taking short rapid breaths for fear of pain from more movement. Everything is worse from movement, and from the slightest touch, for any warmth or heat (except local pain, which is better for hot compresses), for any change of weather (especially from cold to warm) or for movement from a cold to a warm atmosphere.

The remedy also acts on extreme dryness of the mucous membranes and sinovial fluids, (the fluids which lubricate the joints). The patient may be constipated or have a dry hard stool, will have a dry, racking, irritating painful cough, (worse for movement and warm rooms) and will be extremely thirsty for long drinks of cold water at intervals. Colds go to the chest quickly.

The dryness of the sinovial fluid may lead to rheumatic and joint pain: there are stitching tearing pains with swelling. These may be better for rest and pressure, tight bandaging; worse for movement. The pain is so bad that the sufferer wants to move for relief but movement actually makes it worse.

Dryness is also present in the digestive system, which is easily disturbed. There is an unpleasant, bitter taste in the mouth, the tongue has a white/yellow coating; stomach fluids dry up and food lies like a stone. Nausea and vomiting are common. The sufferer craves ice-cold water but usually gets more relief from drinking warm drinks. There is constipation with large, hard, dry, crumbly stools passed with difficulty.

Symptoms tend to be right-sided. Headache accompanies almost all illnesses and vertigo is common. In general, *Bryonia* illnesses develop slowly and insidiously over days; may come on a day or two after exposure. The patient feels very sore, weary and bruised.

Better: for firm pressure, lying on or binding up the painful part, lying motionless, cool atmosphere, cold, cold drinks, cold applications, free perspiration.

Worse: from even the slightest movement, touch, warmth of any kind, 3 a.m., 9 p.m., change of temperature from cold to warm, or from warm to cold as getting chilled when overheated; exposure to dry cold, especially cold east winds.

The person needing *Bryonia* is **irritable** and **worse** for the **slightest movement** therefore better for **pressure**. There is extreme **dryness** and **thirst for long drinks of cold water at intervals.** Symptoms are **worse** from **warmth** and **heat** and also from **cold dry winds.**

This remedy may be indicated in appendicitis, breast milk problems, bronchitis, constipation, coughs and colds, headache, mastitis, meningitis, migraine, muscle and joint pain, nausea and vomiting, vertigo.

Calcarea carbonica
(Calcium carbonate)

This form of calcium is derived from the inside of an oyster shell, and there is no better metaphor for the state of *Calcarea carbonica* which has a vulnerable soft inside protected by a self-grown shell.

In its physical state *Calc carb* is soft, flabby, cold and damp like an oyster. A person needing *Calc carb* will tend to be overweight with flabby muscles and relaxed tissues: she seems boneless. She will be very chilly (though children are often hot), extremely sensitive to cold air, raw winds, draught, storm. Different parts of her can be cold, she can have cold feet and a hot head. She gets a lot of colds which go to the chest. She is also damp: she sweats in spots, in various places, head, forehead, back of neck, front of chest, feet. She has cold clammy hands and a wet fish hand-shake.

There is an inertia about *Calc carb*; the person needing it will be inclined to be slow and lethargic, easily out of breath. Often this is because of glandular inactivity: the pituitary and thyroid glands malfunction. Even mild exertion easily tires her: she gets weak and exhausted mentally and physically and has to give up whatever she is doing. She gets fevers, headaches, heavy sweating after exertion.

Psychologically and emotionally the subject is also rather oyster-like. Soft and vulnerable inside, she experiences terrible anxiety and fear. She is particularly fearful of what people think about her; she is very self-conscious, hates being looked at or laughed at and has a deep fear that people will think she is insane. She is afraid of disease, insects, heights, thunderstorms, insanity, poverty, open spaces, closed spaces, people, the dark and being on her own.

Because she is unsure of herself and how she will be received she can try very hard: she is conscientious, hard-working and methodical because she doesn't really know how to cut corners. She can easily work too hard and tire herself, then she will give up, get depressed and discouraged. She is not directly aggressive but one of her main characteristics is extreme obstinacy. This is how she defends herself against those quicker and cleverer than she is. When in doubt she shuts up and closes down like an oyster, becoming completely unresponsive in order to conceal her internal anxiety.

As in most homoeopathic remedies an opposite state can be found in the picture. A state of oversensitivity can also exist. The person can be jumpy, easily startled at the least noise, exceedingly distressed at hearing of cruelty, scared at the sight of wounds, have an impulse to scream or cry without apparent reason. Her sleep can be disturbed by terrifying dreams; she often has difficulty going to sleep because of a flow of anxious thoughts; she can lie awake till 2, 3, or 4 a.m. This state is seen most clearly in children, but it is the underlying state in the adult and it is her awareness of it that makes her fear insanity.

Children are chubby and round-faced with big bellies; teeth come late and fontanelles stay open a long time; they sweat profusely around the head especially at night, wetting the pillow. They may appear lethargic and be slow to develop. Teething can bring problems. They have frequent colds and recurrent earache. Children can also be hyperactive, restless and bad-tempered with tantrums and convulsions. It is indicated in food-sensitive/allergic children.

Food metabolism is slow and she puts on weight easily, but she is often hungry and desires indigestible things: raw potatoes, coal, pencils, chalk, clay. She also craves sweets, salt, eggs, ice cream, milk, cheese and bread and is sometimes averse to milk, cheese, eggs, meat, fat, coffee. Her food cravings reflect the calcium imbalance present in the system.

Other characteristic symptoms are that she feels fine when constipated, has no urging. The glands are frequently involved and the lymph nodes become hard, inflamed and sore. The remedy has a sour smell; there is sour vomiting, diarrhoea, smell of body, breath etc.

Better: dry weather, constipation, heat, lying down.

Worse: cold of all kinds, cold wet weather, cold water, cold baths, damp, draughts, physical or mental exertion, fresh air, full moon.

The person who needs *Calcarea carbonica* is likely to be **weak** and **easily tired** with **flabby tissues**. She **sweats easily,** is **very chilly** and **sensitive to cold** and **damp.** She is **anxious** and **fearful** especially about what people think of her and **lacks self-confidence** but she can be very **conscientious,** determined and **obstinate.** She has a **slow metabolism, glands** underfunction. She may **crave** or **hate eggs, milk, cheese.** There is also sometimes a **hyperactive** state especially in sleep or in children when the patient is **jumpy,** restless and **easily startled.**

This remedy may be indicated in allergy, anxiety, asthma, boils, colds, convulsions, digestive problems, ear infections, food sensitivity, gallstones, glandular problems, hyperactivity, menopause, mumps, muscle and joint pains, piles, teething, tonsillitis (chronic), toothache, vaginitis, varicose veins.

Causticum
(Potassium hydrate)

A state of paralysis is characteristic of this remedy – a progressive, slow-acting chronic state encompassing paralysis (with weakness and tremor), rheumatism and arthritis. There's a state of lassitude and mental fatigue. The paralysis reaches right through to the emotional layers as well. Anxiety and fear are prominent, paralysing anxiety and fear, worse at twilight and night. There is also a sort of paralysis of confidence and will. The person is extremely cautious and anxious; she can even become suicidal from thinking about anxiety and fears, frighten herself to death. She is full of foreboding and apprehension, jumps at the least noise, has fearful fancies in the dark. Night is a very bad time and there are fears on waking. There are fears of many things: dogs, evil, ghosts, the future. Children do not want to go to bed alone.

People needing this remedy are very sensitive to others: deeply concerned about injustice (especially children). They have intense sympathy with people or animals in pain or in trouble, are almost excessively compassionate. Their anxiety for others is marked. As a defence they can often be very caustic or sarcastic; they can be censorious and critical and are inclined to contradict others. A blustering anger is often present which doesn't last; the person can be quarrelsome and peevish and get incensed at trifles. This is the opposite side to that of the extreme anxiety, lack of self-confidence and timidity.

Pessimism, depression and anxiety are expressed in sudden tears and floods of emotion. They may have a history of suffering from long-lasting grief which has worn them out. A woman needing this remedy may become hopeless, despondent, want to die. She can become conscience-stricken as if she had committed some crime; she may become suspicious of others too. She worries a lot, always having to go back and check whether she has remembered to do something.

The remedy is particularly suited to people with a worn-out constitution who suffer from stiff joints and chronic rheumatic problems causing contraction of the tendons and deformities around the joints. The pains are burning, drawing, sore, raw, with cramps here and there: they are generally worse for cold dry weather and better for wet mild weather. There is restlessness of the legs in bed at night.

There is paralysis of single parts of the body: this may be the result of deep-seated nervous diseases (e.g. Parkinson's) or the acute result of exposure to cold or trauma (e.g. Bell's Palsy). There can be small paralyses of the throat with difficulty swallowing, of the eyelid, causing drooping. Headaches with facial neuralgia are common. The right side is particularly affected.

Very chilly people subject to vertigo which is worse when lying down in bed.

A burning, raw, scraped pain is characteristic and is experienced particularly in sore throats with hoarseness (worse morning), cystitis with acute sensitivity to cold and in the effects of burns and scalds.

Incontinence of urine is an important symptom, worse for coughing, sneezing or exertion. It is caused by muscular weakness or paralysis after childbirth, surgery. There may also be constipation and faecal incontinence arising from weakness of muscles.

Better: cold drinks, damp wet weather, washing, warmth of bed.

Worse: dry, cold or raw air, winds, draughts, extremes of temperature, fats, 3-4 a.m. or evening, change of weather, darkness, burns, fright, grief.

Causticum is characteristically **anxious** and **cautious, worn out** and **worried**. **Sympathetic** to others but often **caustic** and **critical**. They are **chilly** with **raw, burning pains** better for **warm wet weather** and much **worse** for **cold dry weather**. **Incontinence** with **cough** is an important guiding symptom. **Paralysis** and **rheumatic** pain are common in the remedy.

If the general symptoms agree this remedy may be considered in anxiety, Bell's Palsy, burns, cramp, cystitis, grief, incontinence, muscle and joint pain, neuralgia, restless legs, stiff neck, vertigo and dizziness.

Chamomilla
(Chamomile, Corn feverfew)

Sensitivity to pain is the most marked characteristic feature of *Chamomilla*. Wherever the pain is and whatever its cause, it is completely unbearable. It enrages the sufferer and nothing can pacify her. *Chamomilla* is also probably the most irritable remedy in the *Materia Medica*. She is irritable because nothing is right: whatever you do for her it won't be the right thing. She is easily offended, becomes melancholy and refuses to reply when spoken to. She is irritable if spoken to or looked at. She is angry and irritable with or because of pain. A lot of complaints are caused by or associated with anger. She is extremely restless with anger and pain, paces about to relieve it.

The uninhibited expression of anger and pain is more likely to be seen to its fullest extent in children and so this remedy is highly indicated in many children's complaints (see chapter 8). However, it may also be indicated for adults driven beyond normal restraint by the intensity of their pain.

It can often be helpful in gynaecological conditions, where pain is frequently unbearable. The woman's breasts can be very tender and the nipples inflamed. She will be irritable before periods. She may have severe pain during a period, haemorrhages of dark blood with labour-like pains. It may be indicated in threatened miscarriage if there is unbearable pain from the back to the middle of the thighs. It is useful for the severe pains of labour.

When there is pain in the muscles and joints the pains drive the sufferer from the bed to walk the floor; she is thirsty, hot and beside herself with anguish. She may have cramps in the legs.

She has very little appetite but there may be a craving for or aversion to coffee or narcotics. There is a marked thirst for cold water, desire for acid drinks. The sufferer is prone to attacks of severe vomiting with retching; she is bilious from anger. She may have slimy diarrhoea.

Sleep is characteristically disturbed and restless. Nightmares are common. She is inclined to get hot in bed, throw the bedclothes off and stick her feet out. She sweats easily and is better for sweat. She is extremely sensitive to wind, chill from cold damp air and cold.

Better: being carried, or riding in the car, heat (except toothache), warm humid weather.

Worse: draughts, wind, wet, getting angry, 9 p.m. to midnight, coffee, narcotics, before and during periods.

Chamomilla is needed by people who are **excitable** and **hypersensitive** both physically and emotionally. They are extremely **sensitive** to **pain** which is **intolerable.** They are also easily offended, **irritable, angry** and **quarrelsome. Restlessness, temper tantrums** and **rage** are prominent in its picture. They are **better** for **being carried, worse night,** 9 p.m.-**midnight.** They are strongly affected by **wind** and **cold.**

The remedy may be indicated in the following conditions: colic, earache, food sensitivity, labour pains, period pain, muscle and joint pains, sciatica, teething, toothache.

China
(Cinchona, Peruvian bark)

The woman who needs *China* is exhausted, edgy, irritable, touchy, apathetic, disinclined to make any intellectual effort. She doesn't want company or activity, is very sensitive to noise. Frequently this state will have been brought about by illness, especially by prolonged mental and physical strain or by conditions involving exhausting discharges and loss of fluids: prolonged breast feeding, heavy bleeding, diarrhoea and vomiting or excessive sweating, for instance.

She might become temporarily anaemic and look very pale with dark circles around the eyes. She will have no vitality, may feel faint and suffer from ringing in the ears with sweating on exertion and during sleep.

Timidity and anxiety are strong: the woman is full of fears especially at night, she is particularly afraid of dogs and crawling insects. She expects to be criticized and imagines that people do so. She can even feel suicidal but lacks the energy or motivation to act.

She is very chilly and sensitive to cold and draughts, worse for cold weather and fresh air. She has a tendency to flushes of heat and bouts of shivering. Her senses generally are very acute: she is sensitive to noise and external impressions. She suffers from cutting, tearing neuralgic pains that are better from hard pressure and worse for light touch; headache is worse when she combs her hair, for example. Severe cutting tearing pains in labour.

An important general symptom is that things affect her periodically: every other day or at the same time every day.

She can be feverish with severe chills; alternate bouts of sweating and shivering, thirst before the chill, absence of thirst during hot stage, unquenchable thirst during sweats.

Her digestive problems are related to the gall bladder or the bowels. She has a great deal of bloating, gas and distension which is not better for belching or flatus (unlike *Carbo veg*). She suffers from painless watery diarrhoea causing extreme weakness. Green watery corroding stools, with colic, thirst, bitter taste and bitter belching. She is hungry but quickly feels full; craves condiments, stimulants, alcohol. She is averse to butter and fatty foods; intolerant of sour things, fish, fruit, wine and milk. She gets diarrhoea after milk and fruit (especially infants).

It is a haemorrhagic remedy: the patient suffers from frequent nosebleeds. Periods tend to be early and heavy with dark clotted blood. There may be haemorrhaging during pregnancy, a profuse discharge of dark blood with labour pains. It is indicated in bleeding anywhere, particularly when accompanied by buzzing in the ears and general weakness.

She is sleepy during the day but cannot sleep at night; restless especially early at night. Vivid distressing dreams interrupt sleep.

Better: firm pressure, warmth, sleep.

Worse: slight touch, draughts, cold, fresh air, movement, night (especially midnight), autumn, periodically, eating fruit or acid things.

China is **touchy, irritable, exhausted** and **depleted** from **loss of body fluids.**

If the general symptoms agree, it may be indicated in diarrhoea, gallstones, gastroenteritis, low blood pressure with dizziness, pounding headaches, ringing in the ears, tinnitus, Ménière's disease.

Cimicifuga, also called Actaea racemosa (Black snake root, Black cohosh)

This is a remedy that is useful in a great many women's complaints, but it is not as well known as it should be.

The woman needing it is gloomy and morose, she has a strong

sensation of a heavy cloud descending on her. She can suffer great depression with dreams of impending evil. She has all sorts of terrible fears, is afraid that something is going to happen, that she is going to die, that she will be poisoned or that she will go insane. She can talk incessantly, changing from one subject to another like *Lachesis* and she is nervous, fidgety and excitable. She sighs a lot.

She is markedly chilly and generally worse for the cold. Pains are often neuralgic, shooting pains: the top of her head feels as if it might fly off and she has shooting pains in her eyes.

She suffers from some pre-menstrual tension but the worst time for her is during the periods. All her symptoms are worse then: the greater the flow, the greater the pain. The flow is characteristically heavy, dark, coagulated, offensive, she has backache. She suffers from sharp labour-like abdominal pains which make her double up. Between periods she is exhausted. They are always irregular. In the menopause these symptoms may be exaggerated: she may have flooding, flushing, headaches (terrible migraines) and severe mental depression.

Her anxiety level is particularly strong in pregnancy (not without reason, as she has a tendency to miscarry). She suffers from shooting, flying pains during the later months and sore bruised pains in the joints and lower back. She has nausea and vomiting in pregnancy.

Labour is also a difficult experience: her whole body feels sore and bruised and sensitive to touch, she has shooting flying pains. Labour is weak rather like *Caulophyllum*, or spasmodic with faintness or cramps. There are afterpains with great sensitiveness and intolerance of pain: nausea and vomiting.

The remedy may be highly indicated after childbirth when the loquacious and agitated depression may get very strong. She may feel suicidal or want to kill the baby.

The remedy's other main area of usefulness is in rheumatic pain: there is stiffness and pain in the neck as if her head were pulled backwards. The rheumatic pains are worse in the cold damp weather, worse at night and when associated with menstrual problems. They tend to shoot downwards.

Better: warmth, open air, pressure, continued motion.

Worse: damp, cold, during periods.

Cimicifuga is **severely depressed** and **loquacious,** is **chilly,** has **rheumatic** and **neuralgic pain** and everything is **worse during periods** and **labour.**

If the general symptoms agree, it may be indicated in afterpains, headaches and migraine, labour, morning sickness, muscle and joint pain, period pain, post-natal depression, stiff neck.

Gelsemium
(Yellow jasmine, Wild woodbine)

There is a state of relaxation and weakness which is almost paralysis associated with *Gelsemium*. It also has an extremely anxious state: anyone needing it will be very apprehensive about everything: death, crowds, wide open spaces, falling, exams, public appearances. In anxiety she will tremble, seize up, become paralysed, heavy and sluggish, she may be unable to speak, she may get diarrhoea. She is also worse for mental exertion, afraid of public speaking or even having company present. Complaints may follow fear, shock, embarrassment or fright. Also can be ill from over-excitement.

There is a sluggish depression associated with the remedy. The sufferer wants to be left alone, wants to be quiet, but at the same time hates isolation. Depression typically comes on after receiving bad news; finds it difficult to talk about emotions.

People who need *Gelsemium* are intensely weary. Their bodies feel heavy (arms and legs feel like lead). They are trembly from exhaustion and worse for any extra exertion, physical or mental. A feeling of great weight and tiredness runs through the remedy, they are so weary and heavy that they must lie down and be still. They tremble if they attempt to move. Just as the jasmine plant needs to be supported on a frame or it would collapse, so the person needing *Gelsemium* wilts and collapses.

It is most often associated with the extreme weakness of flu but also good in cases of nervous prostration or nervous excitement, especially when the bowels are loose and there is nervous diarrhoea or frequent urination. The remedy is well indicated wherever the state contains a sort of paralysis.

The fever associated with *Gelsemium* is usually of gradual onset, may take days to develop. The patient is very cold with chills running up and down the back. The patient keeps as still as does the one needing *Bryonia* but out of tiredness and weariness, not from pain. She has profuse exhaustive sweats but is too weak to move. The limbs are heavy. She is thirstless, has a flushed, mottled dusky red or purple face with half-closed eyes, cold extremities, is dazed and delirious. It is the most important of flu remedies, especially for flu that comes on gradually in mild damp weather.

Complaints which come and go gradually and hang round, tiring the patient and proving difficult to shake off are characteristic. It has slow congestive complaints.

Blurred vision is a very marked characteristic of *Gelsemium* whatever the associated complaint, especially with the characteristic congestive headaches with violent pain at the back and bottom of the head.

Better: urination, sweating, movement.

Worse: heat, hot weather, bad news, excitement, anticipation, getting cold after overheating, physical exertion.

Gelsemium is **anxious, timid, trembling, weary, weak** and almost **paralysed** with **fright, emotion.**

This remedy is well indicated in anticipatory anxiety, colds, fevers, flu, M.E., nervous diarrhoea, exam fears, nervousness generally.

Hepar sulphuris calcareum
(calcium sulphide: flowers of sulphur + inner part of oyster shells)

Psychological and physical oversensitivity runs through this remedy. Emotionally the sufferers are touchy, oversensitive, irritable, impatient, discontented and quarrelsome and they are physically oversensitive to impressions, touch, surroundings, pain, cold. They may faint from pain. Any infected part is extremely tender to touch and the slightest pressure causes a sharp pain, as though there were a splinter pushing into the affected place. When ill in bed they cannot bear even the bedclothes to touch them; they are sensitive to breaths of air, to the least draught, to putting even a hand outside the bedclothes. This extreme sensitivity of the part to touch is one of the most characteristic symptoms of the remedy.

Suppuration is also a prominent feature: everything festers and suppurates. Everywhere feels sore and bruised as if there were a boil there. Psychologically also the sufferers might be described as suppurating: they are hasty and impulsive: ready to burst out. They can be angry and abusive, volcanic. At times they have an impulse to commit suicide.

Catarrhal states are also prominent. There are colds which start with an itchy throat with a lot of sneezing and obstruction every time they go into a cold wind. The discharge is initially watery, later thick, yellow and offensive, smelling often like decomposed cheese. Face aches, bones are sore to touch. *Hepar sulph* usually comes in when a cold has reached the ripe stage and phlegm has formed. Splintering pains in throat or a sensation as if a fish bone were in the throat are characteristic. Throat is worse for swallowing, ear can hurt on swallowing. If cold goes to chest *Hepar* may avert or improve bronchitis.

All complaints are worse for cold, dry cold and better in warm wet weather. (*Silica* is worse in wet cold and better in warm dry).

Patients want warm rooms and to be well covered. The least uncovering causes chilliness or cough.

Indicated in neuralgia, particularly right side of face, after *Belladonna*, seemingly indicated, has failed, especially after exposure to cold winds.

There are thick yellow cheesy discharges: all discharges smell sour or of decomposed cheese. There are sour offensive sweats.

Better: Eating a meal, staying in the warm, applying compresses and wrapping the head up.

Worse: Cold air and draughts, undressing and touching affected parts, morning, lying on painful side, touch, pressure, motions, exertion, tight clothing.

Hepar sulph is **impulsive, over-sensitive,** greatly affected by **pain, worse** for **touch, draught, cold. Suppuration** with **splinter-like pains** and **yellow cheesy sour-smelling discharges** are characteristic.

The remedy is strongly indicated wherever there is pus, especially where it has formed rapidly: abscesses, boils, conjunctivitis, croup, ear infections, <u>tonsillitis</u>, whitlows. It is also indicated in bronchitis, catarrh, irritability, neuralgia, sinusitis.

Ignatia amara
(Strychnos ignatia; St Ignatius' bean)

The *Ignatia* state is highly emotional, changeable and unstable. The sufferer can be sad and tearful and has a tendency to brood over thoughts and problems. She cries easily but can laugh just as easily or laugh till she cries; laughing and joking are strongly marked symptoms. She may burst out in anger and then suppress it. Any condition brought on by (or accompanied by) emotional stress, grief, fear, anger, disappointed love, embarrassment or being criticized may respond to *Ignatia*. She is more reserved than *Pulsatilla*, less so than *Nat mur*: she does not resent sympathy and consolation.

It is the first remedy to think of in states of grief and distress or whenever emotional balance is lost. The woman is quite reserved in character like *Nat mur* and she tries to hide her deep emotions but they break out. She is more extrovert than *Nat mur,* more impulsive, excitable and headstrong.

The patient is generally oversensitive to excitement, pain and smells, especially tobacco. She faints easily and sighs a great deal. Deep sighing is very characteristic.

There are contradictory and paradoxical symptoms: the sufferer is moody, laughs and cries alternately; is both reserved and over-expressive; digests heavy and indigestible food better than light food and experiences a nervous hunger which is not improved by eating: the more she eats the more she wants; throat pain is better for swallowing solids, worse for swallowing liquids; stomach ache and nausea is better for eating, eating causes hunger. She craves indigestible things, like fruit, sour and acidic foods and unusual foods when ill.

The remedy is very spasmodic in nature: sudden fleeting pains show up in various places, there are spasms and tics in the face and eyelids; breathing, coughing and period pains are all spasmodic. There are severe, cramping, labour-like period pains with heavy bleeding and clotting.

A feeling of a lump in the throat is characteristic. Headache feels as if a nail were being driven through the side or back of the head. She suffers from constipation from emotion.

Better: heat; eating, firm pressure.

Worse: emotional shock, fear, fright, worry, bereavement, apprehension, suppressing grief or other emotions, morning 11 a.m., strong smells (tobacco, coffee etc.), pressure on the painless side, fresh air.

Ignatia is **paradoxical, emotional** and **excitable.** There is a **spasmodic** tendency, both psychological, with nervousness, sharp outbreaks of **anger,** intense **laughing** and **crying** spells and a good deal of **sighing,** and physical, with spasmodic **yawning, twitching,** jerking, sudden fleeting erratic pains.

It may be indicated for the effects of any emotion, especially grief, headache, indigestion, period pains, shock, spasm.

Ipecacuanha (Cephaelis ipecacuanha)

This remedy is most useful in acute situations where there is nausea, difficult breathing or haemorrhaging. All complaints are accompanied by nausea. Bleeding is frequent: oozing with intermittent gushes of bright red blood. The remedy has a very chilly and usually thirstless picture. There are sporadic patches of exhaustion and prostration. The mood may be peevish, irritable, impatient and scornful. Hard to please.

The cough is dry, teasing, spasmodic and suffocative, accompanied by nausea and vomiting. It is worse for movement and being outside, better for rest and heat. Coughing is often accompanied by nosebleeds or bleeding from the lungs. A lot of mucus lies in the bronchial tubes and lungs and there is wheezing, rattling and gagging. However, the cough remains active, even violent. The sufferer has to sit up to breathe, needs oxygen. It is indicated in moist asthma. Incessant violent cough with nosebleeds suggests this remedy in whooping cough. It is indicated in bronchitis in old people when the condition is worse for damp or sudden change in weather.

There are occipital (base of skull) headaches accompanied by nausea, neuralgic pains in the eye.

All symptoms are accompanied by severe nausea with a clean or slightly coated tongue and a great deal of salivation. It is indicated in persistent violent nausea which is not relieved by vomiting. Feels disgust for all types of food.

There is painful diarrhoea: stools yellow/green with nausea and colic, griping. Autumnal diarrhoea caused by eating unripe fruit or when the weather begins to turn cold. There is a strong desire for sweets which can cause the characteristic green slimy diarrhoea.

Periods are too early and too frequent, there is bright red clotted blood with faintness. There may be bleeding between periods: bright red, gushing, worse for movement. In pregnancy there will be terrible nausea, probably with excessive salivation. There may be profuse bleeding during and after labour.

Better: Firm pressure, open air, at rest.

Worse: Cold weather, excessive heat, damp weather, veal, pork, ices.

The characteristics of Ipecac are **persistent nausea** with **vomiting** and excess **saliva, bright red blood** and **difficult breathing**.

It may be indicated in asthma, bronchitis, colitis, conjunctivitis, diarrhoea, hay fever, haemorrhage, headaches, heavy periods, migraine, morning sickness, nosebleeds, toothache, travel sickness, sea sickness, whooping cough.

Kali carbonicum
(Potassium carbonate)

Weariness and tiredness run through this remedy. It is a 'born tired' sort of person who always seems drowsy and yawns a lot. She will fall asleep, especially after eating and sometimes even over food. She is easily exhausted and worse for any exertion, mental or physical. She may look flabby and a bit waterlogged. A lot of the symptoms are connected with the digestive system. The state is very like that of hypoglycaemia (low blood sugar).

Everything is affected by weariness. The muscles are very weak, especially the back muscles and the woman will frequently suffer from low back pain: her back is always 'giving out'. The ligaments around the joints lose their elasticity and power. The heart muscle can also be weak. There may be lassitude, weariness and heaviness of the extremities. In advanced stages of illness, paralysis can even set in.

Pains are described as stitching and can occur anywhere. They are worse for rest or motion and when lying on the affected side. They are particularly noticeable in labour where labour is too weak. They are also characteristic in arthritic pain.

The digestive system is deeply implicated in any illness. Subjects have trouble with flatulence, distension and constipation. Food is often repugnant to them; they suffer from sour belching and acid risings and a strange empty feeling in the pit of the stomach. They crave sweets, sugar and starchy foods. They are worse for missing a meal but also worse for eating, especially hot food; there is often sensitivity to various foods. Anxiety is felt in the stomach.

Periods are profuse and exhausting; there may be a long cycle.

Kali carb is one of the coldest remedies there is. The woman is very sensitive to the cold, to draughts and cold air. She is much worse in the cold; better for warmth but worse for being overheated. She is very susceptible to damp.

There is a tendency to catch colds and a general severely catarrhal state. Nasal catarrh spreads quickly down throat leading to bronchitis and pneumonia if it is not checked. Hard white mucus comes up and flies out of the mouth when coughing.

The kidneys are weak and there is a general waterlogged state. She may be flabby, retaining fluids easily and tending to overweight. A characteristic feature is swelling of the upper eyelids. She is also sweaty, sweats from the slightest exertion. All symptoms appear predominantly on the right side.

A sensitive nervous system makes the subjects easily frightened, of dogs, the dark, the future. They want company for fear of being alone. They are very anxious and apprehensive, worrying about everything, poverty, death, the future, especially their health. They experience the anxiety in the pit of the stomach. They feel anxious when hungry. They are also very timid and apprehensive and unlikely to confront directly. They are nervy and irritable, 'highly strung' and 'uptight', easily aggravated by noise and disorder. As with *Causticum*, the anxiety is founded on a lack of self-confidence and a sensitivity of the nervous system. They are easily startled. They either can't sleep or wake between 2 and 5 a.m.; sleep is full of disturbing dreams. She may become absent-minded and take to constantly misplacing things, making mistakes, missing words out. She can then become a prey to feelings of failure and melancholia.

It is hard to get a good symptom picture from a person needing *Kali carb*. She will understate her emotions and attempt to explain, indeed over-explain, everything. She may be impatient of considering matters in ways other than the ones she has already thought through, taking refuge in 'knowing what's right' to support herself in uncertainty.

Better: getting warm, open air, sitting bent, warmth of any kind.

Worse: in morning 2-5 a.m., cold, chill, damp, pain worse lying on affected side, pressure, fast movement, open air, any exertion, especially sexual, during periods, during and after eating, missed periods, getting too hot.

The *Kali carb* state is one of **weariness** and **tiredness. Everything affects the stomach,** there is **low back pain,** marked **sweating** and **catarrh.** The sufferer is **anxious** and **apprehensive, worse 2-5 a.m.** and **cold. Right sided** complaints and **stitching pains** are characteristic.

It may be indicated in allergy (especially to food), asthma, backache, bronchitis, catarrh, gall bladder colic, hypoglycaemia, indigestion, labour pains, after-effects of labour, menopause problems, muscle and joint pain, period problems, tonsillitis.

Lachesis (Lachesis trigonocephalus)
(Venom of the Surukuku or Bushmaster snake)

This snake venom has a powerful effect on the nervous system, causing stimulation and increased activity followed by depression and stagnation. It also affects the blood, causing first clotting and then haemorrhaging, and both are characteristic of the remedy.

A woman who needs *Lachesis* alternates between periods of excitement and periods of depression. The alternation of states can vary from the intensity of the manic depressive to the milder swings of a 'moody' type of person. This cycle can take place daily with, for example, sadness in the morning and excitement in the evening, or there can be more prolonged periods of each state. Sometimes the depression is caused by exhaustion after the energetic state. She is easily exhausted from the slightest exertion, physical or mental, and is worse in the morning or from the heat of the sun. Tiredness is not helped by sleeping.

In one phase of the cycle the woman who needs *Lachesis* will be intense, energetic, self-confident, enthusiastic, excitable and enormously articulate and talkative. She will be full of ideas and conviction, fascinating like a snake. In the other phase of the cycle there will be periods of depression, anxiety and even silence; the talkativeness may become rambling incoherence. Suspiciousness, jealousy and spitefulness may emerge and she will strike like a snake; imagining that she is being cheated, talked about, hated and plotted against, she will strike first.

The unconscious, the shadow, is never far from expression in the *Lachesis* personality. The subjects are often very sensitive, even psychic; they commonly have disturbing dreams of ghosts, the dead, funerals and coffins. Sleeping can feel dangerous because of the release of unconscious material. They are easily affected by alcohol which, again, allows material to erupt from the unconscious. Sexuality is a strongly developed area and if it cannot be expressed there can be problems. *Lachesis* is well and fully functioning as long as she can express herself, discharge her strong feelings, her ideas, her plans. She is ill when this expression is blocked.

A very low self-esteem lies at the root of a lot of *Lachesis* symptoms. The woman needs to be acknowledged as exceptional, as special, and if that cannot be achieved she may be extremely negative and take revenge, behaving maliciously and vindictively. She cannot stand being limited, controlled, constricted.

The physical expressions of *Lachesis* are just as intense. The intolerance of constriction comes through strongly: she cannot stand any constriction of clothing, especially round the throat and abdomen. All symptoms are worse if there is any block to expression. So when periods are suppressed by, for example, the Pill or menopause there can be sleeplessness and headaches. Emotional symptoms are all worse from delayed or suppressed periods; PMS is appalling with anger, jealousy, suspiciousness, which all disappear with the flow of blood. The headaches, characteristically congested and throbbing, are better when a period starts or when there is a nosebleed. Period pains are also congested and spasmodic and better when the flow is established. Colds start by being very stuffed up and are better when they begin to get runny.

The woman easily gets too hot and is much better for being outside in the fresh air, for cold compresses applied to local complaints. She is much worse after sleeping, much worse on waking: everything is worse, cough, headache, pain, mood. Sometimes she even fears going to sleep because she knows she will be worse in the morning. She is also much worse in the spring, a general time of awakening and warmth.

Because of its effects on the blood, *Lachesis* is an important remedy in menstruation. There is likely to be very heavy clotting and bleeding throughout the years of menstruation, and the menopause is a particularly difficult time with haemorrhaging, hot flushes and varicose veins which may ulcerate, throbbing piles which are relieved by bleeding. There is also a tendency to easy bruising and high blood pressure, palpitations and bursting throbbing headaches, even stroke.

The blood is very much involved in other ways: *Lachesis* is a major remedy for septic states, infections and poisoning of the blood. The blood is very visible beneath the skin which goes mottled, purplish when infected. The complexion in general tends to be ruddy or blotchy with visible veins.

The whole body is very sensitive to touch, especially the neck and throat. There is a characteristic sensation of having a lump in the throat (sometimes in the bladder or arm). Light pressure aggravates a sore throat so it is better for swallowing solid food. Swallowing can be difficult, in general, and hot liquids are more difficult to swallow than cold.

The woman may crave coffee, alcohol and oysters. She has a strong dislike of bread and hot drinks though she is generally very thirsty. The remedy tends to have left-sided complaints, or complaints which go from left to right.

Better: discharges e.g. periods, pus, nasal catarrh, verbal diarrhoea; moderate temperatures; fresh air.

Worse: Delayed or suppressed discharges, before periods; being touched, especially round neck and throat; heat of the sun, heat generally; going from cold to warm, becoming warm; left side, Spring; after sleeping on waking, alcohol, tight clothes.

Lachesis has **intense mood swings,** from **sadness** to **excitability,** all the symptoms are **worse after sleep, on waking, worse** on the **left side. Talkativeness, jealousy** and **suspiciousness** are the main psychological indications and there is extreme **oversensitivity** both physical and emotional: the sufferer is **worse** for **light, noise, light touch,** very much **worse** for **heat, craves fresh air.** Cannot bear **emotional constriction** or **constriction round throat** or

abdomen. Subject feels **better** for **discharge** of any kind: body fluids, emotional material.

This remedy may be indicated in abscesses and boils, anxiety and depression, grief, headaches, problems of menstruation, especially during menopause, sore throats, tonsillitis, varicose ulcers.

Lycopodium clavatum
(Wolf's claw, Club moss)

The person who needs *Lycopodium* can appear to be very self-confident and self-reliant. There is a high self-esteem, which is generally well-founded since the person usually works hard and performs well. The subject may have a tendency to be a little too confident, rather irritatingly sure that she is right, often refusing even to discuss a matter under dispute, but this may not seem a very important fault. When this tendency is exaggerated in illness, however, or when it is part of the illness, the woman can become self-righteous, overbearing, even haughty. She may be the kind of person who is agreeable outside the home and tyrannical within it.

The confident air may have been adopted over many years as a cover for insecurity and fear. Often the person may have used her mind, her capacity to understand things, as a means of survival: she has constantly looked for proof, facts and evidence, has had little practice in trusting feelings and intuitions. So, though she seems self-assured, she is driven by insecurity, anxiety and fear of failure. She never feels successful, however well she does. There is a chronic lack of self-confidence with many fears and anxieties, defended against by an air of detachment and superiority. This leads to fears of having to appear in public, or take exams: anticipatory anxiety is enormous for she fears that here, at last, she will be exposed, found out.

She is somewhat emotionally detached, is fearful of letting anyone get too close to her, and yet is afraid of being alone. She likes to be alone but with someone on hand, perhaps in the next room. Paradoxically, she can have a very amorous nature.

She is afraid of crowds, closed places, the dark, death. She has fears about financial security, worries that she will not have enough money to live on. All her fears are related to the ability to be self-sufficient, which is of paramount importance. She copes with the anxiety and fear by working hard, being assertive, taking charge of her environment.

As the years go by or when she gets ill, it may become more difficult to keep up the effort of staying in control; energy runs out and fatigue begins to set in after intellectual exertion. She becomes unable to think clearly, her memory does not work so well, she may spell things incorrectly. Her worst nightmare is fulfilled: she begins to perform inadequately. This can come about as a result of chronic illness, of the menopause or even of premature senility. She may look older than she is, with a yellowish skin and a wrinkled frowning forehead. Her hair can go grey early.

The main physical problems are connected with the (progressively inefficient) functioning of the liver which affects the digestive system. The sufferer feels hungry, eats and feels full and bloated after a few mouthfuls or else eats a huge meal and still feels ravenously hungry. There is a lot of gas and bloating which is worse after eating; she can not stand tight clothing round the abdomen. Her stomach rumbles and gurgles loud enough to be heard and there is often very offensive flatulence which is not relieved by breaking wind or belching. She may have painful indigestion with acid dyspepsia for hours. She may suffer from nausea and vomiting, recurrent bilious attacks. There is a tendency to gallstones and gallstone colic. She may be extremely constipated.

She craves sugar, sweets and oysters which disagree with her; she cannot digest starchy food, onions, cabbage or milk. She is not particularly thirsty but likes drinks to be hot, is worse from cold drinks and coffee. She gets headaches from digestive disturbances, (most often right-sided and above the eye). Headaches are often brought on if a meal is late: they are better for eating, worse from heat, from warmth of the bed and from lying down; better from cold, cool fresh air. All symptoms are worse in late afternoon.

Her chest is also a problem area: colds go to the chest, there is difficult and asthmatic breathing in catarrh of the chest; bronchitis, pneumonia. Troubles have often existed since an attack of bronchitis or pneumonia. Lung problems tend to be right-sided.

Before periods the woman tends to be irritable and depressed and her digestive system will be disturbed. Periods may be absent, late or protracted. Bleeding is profuse. There may be neuralgic pains in the right ovary and dryness of the vagina.

Exhaustion is a marked feature: exhaustion from overwork and stress. There is an exhausted toxic state in which uric acid piles up in the system causing gouty rheumatism and high blood pressure. The eliminative organs can no longer cope and the person eventually loses all vitality, becoming exhausted, dry and withered, appearing old even if not old.

She is very chilly and sensitive to cold though generally better for open air and worse in a warm room. One foot may be hot while the other is cold.

Better: in open air, motion, warm drinks, lying on left side.

Worse: 4 to 8 p.m., from cold air, cold drinks, warm rooms, tight clothing around waist, oysters, cabbage.

The characteristic symptoms of this remedy display a paradoxical picture. **Lack of self confidence** and **haughtiness, timidity** and **rudeness, abusiveness** and **flattery, intellectual ability** and **mental confusion** and **forgetfulness** are all equally present. She is **chilly** but **better** in the **open air. Complaints** tend to be **right-sided** or to move from **right** to **left**; they are **worse** 4-8 p.m. **Flatulence** is marked. Desires **sweet** food and **hot** drinks.

It may be indicated in anticipatory anxiety, chest disorders, constipation, cystitis, flatulence, high blood pressure, indigestion, kidney stones, lack of self-confidence, period pains.

Mercurius solubilis
(Mercury, quicksilver)

The sufferer is full of anxiety, fear and apprehension; hasty, hurried, restless and impulsive. This characteristic may most often probably be seen in nervous children who talk very quickly and are inclined to stutter. They find it difficult to stay still, feel hurried inside. It is appropriate for mischievous, sometimes malicious, children who are always into things, restless, rushing unproductively from one thing to another.

There is also a state of depression and confusion associated with mercury poisoning in which the sufferer is psychologically slow if not actually retarded (either constitutionally, or as a result of accident or age) with a bad memory. Time seems to pass very slowly, they suffer from weariness and disenchantment with life. They have poor comprehension and memory, forgetting names and what they were going to say.

The glands are frequently involved in mercurial illness: there can be swollen glands anywhere, but the salivary glands and the glands in the throat and neck are particularly commonly involved.

Pus formation is also characteristic of the remedy: infections and wounds suppurate rapidly with burning and stinging. In chicken pox the patient develops large pussy eruptions that become open sores. There can be chronic conjunctivitis, repeated ear infections with offensive pussy discharges, breast abscesses, abscesses which form in the glands and at the roots of the teeth. Yellow or yellowy-green pussy burning discharges are characteristic.

There is also a great deal of ulceration, especially of the mucous membranes as in mouth ulcers, stomach ulcers and colitis.

Many symptoms of *Merc sol* are expressed in the mouth and throat. Sufferers have foul-smelling breath, spongy, yellow-white gums which tend to ulcerate, general redness and ulceration of the mouth and throat with swollen glands. The tongue has a thick yellowish coating; it is swollen and shows the marks of teeth on its sides. There is often a metallic or sweet or salty taste and a sense of dryness with intense thirst. Gums are often swollen. There is increased saliva.

The person needing this remedy will be both hungry and thirsty. There is an insatiable hunger but an aversion to meat, fat and butter and stomach upsets from eating sweets. There is a burning thirst for cold drinks, especially milk and beer. Indigestion is common in pregnancy.

There can be bad leucorrhoea or thrush, worse at night with the characteristic burning yellowy green and bloody discharge, with a sensation of rawness. Itching and burning are relieved by washing with cold water. Periods tend to be heavy. A characteristic feature is the presence of milk in the breasts during periods or in non-pregnant women. If there is morning sickness it is accompanied by profuse salivation. Perspiration is profuse and smelly.

Better: moderate temperatures.

Worse: almost everything, especially night, extremes of temperature, change of temperature, sweating. Right-sided.

The characteristic symptoms of this remedy are **inflammation** with **pus formation** usually accompanied by **swollen lymph nodes/glands**. There will usually be **profuse smelly perspiration** and enormously **increased saliva.** The person may be **trembling** and will be **worse** at **night.** The person is **sensitive** to **changes** of **temperature, worse** for **heat** in any form and from **cold damp** air.

If the general symptoms agree this remedy should be considered in the following conditions: chicken pox, colitis, cystitis, ear infections, leucorrhoea, morning sickness, mouth ulcers, mumps, ovaritis, rheumatism, sore throats, thrush, tonsillitis, urethritis.

Natrum muriaticum
(Sodium chloride)

The tendency to hold on to things runs through both physical and emotional states in this remedy. A woman needing it will hold on to her emotions, appearing very reserved, closed and introverted. Her body will hold on to fluids so that, for instance, periods begin late in puberty, there may be loss of periods altogether, bloating before periods, pre-menstrual headaches from water retention.

The woman who needs *Nat mur* will appear to be very quiet and self-contained. She will be perfectly pleasant but slightly on guard and will give very little away about herself: she is intent on avoiding emotional entanglement with others. Nevertheless she is easy to talk to, a good listener, sympathetic to others.

A woman needing *Nat mur* will often not be aware of her own feelings at all. Having dealt with them over the years by burying and ignoring them or keeping them to herself, she no longer has free access to them and often can only get in touch with this side of herself when alone. She can cry and grieve when alone. She cannot share feelings: it is too dangerous, she might get hurt. She does not let anyone see her cry: if she cries she cries alone and does not like sympathy or consolation because she does not believe it is genuine or that people really understand. She prefers to be alone, especially when there is any possibility of becoming emotional or out of control. If she does come to trust someone, however, that relationship becomes extremely important.

Emotions are very strong, even though they are rarely expressed satisfactorily. They run very deep and the control of them dominates her life. One of her greatest fears and anxieties is that she will be robbed: it is a fear of having something taken from her without her permission, of being broken into. Emotions may leak out despite herself, she may laugh uncontrollably at something sad or serious, cry while laughing or cry a great deal over what appear to others to be trifles. She may be cheerful and sad in quick alternation. She may overreact to a small thing and get suddenly and surprisingly angry though she has not responded to many apparently worse things.

The past is important. Her emotional life is lived in the past. She finds it difficult, if not impossible, to let go of disappointments or hurts. If she has had a broken love affair in the past the sense of loss and betrayal will persist; if she has had a bereavement she will find it difficult to resolve the grief. She is haunted by unpleasant thoughts about the past, about how she has been wronged. She bears grudges against anyone who has offended her, even to the point of planning revenge. However, she will say nothing about it either to that person or to others.

She is very fearful and has many complaints from fright. She also descends into deep depression from time to time, often too deep for her to be able to acknowledge the despair. The desire for death and a loathing of life is a very strong symptom, though it seems to remain passive: suicide or suicidal thoughts are not present.

Much of the suppressed emotion finds an outlet and expression through the body in illness or fear of illness which would be the ultimate loss of self-control.

Fluid imbalance is marked in the physical symptoms. *Natrum mur* shows either great dryness of the mucous membranes, like *Bryonia*, or else retains large amounts of fluid, holding on to water as to tears. There is dryness of the mouth, throat, rectum and vagina. Loss of blood during periods may be so heavy as to lead to anaemia. The mucous membranes and skin may be very dry or may produce thick, white or clear watery burning discharges.

The woman may be thin and poorly nourished. She gets thin even while eating well. It is as if really taking anything in or digesting anything is impossible. She actually feels better on an empty stomach. She gets easily exhausted. She has a craving for (or an aversion to) bread and salt. She is thirsty for large quantities of water.

Colds and flu characteristically begin with sneezing and a watery nasal discharge (or one like raw egg white), then progress to a blocked nose. Cold sores are a marked feature along with dry mouth and lips and a sometimes bitter taste. The remedy is frequently well indicated in chronic nasal allergies.

The time of menstruation is an important one. There can be early difficulty in establishing periods and later periods may be scanty, delayed or absent altogether. Pre-menstrually there is fluid retention, swollen breasts, the woman is depressed and irritable, feeling weary and weak and being prone to headaches. There is a tendency to vaginal thrush, dryness, and pain during intercourse because of dryness.

Better: open air, cool bathing, sweating, rest, going without regular meals, tight clothing, rubbing, lying on right side, seashore.

Worse: 9-11 a.m., with the sun, summer, dampness, mental exertion, violent emotions; sympathy, puberty, bread, fat, acid food, seashore, noise, music, touch, pressure, full moon.

The most characteristic symptom of *Natrum muriaticum* is **emotional reserve** and **introversion**. She likes being **alone,** is **worse** for **sympathy** and **company** yet is herself **sympathetic** to others. She suffers from the long-term effects of **grief. Fluid retention** is also strong in the remedy. A general **dryness** runs through the remedy, though her face can be greasy; she is markedly **thirsty.** She is **easily startled, craves** (or is **averse** to) salt, salty foods and bread. **Cold sores** are characteristic and a crack often forms in the middle of the bottom lip.

This remedy may be indicated in anaemia, anorexia, anxiety, cold sores, runny colds, depression, fear, grief, headaches, herpes, late-starting periods, PMS, allergic rhinitis, involuntary urination, water retention.

Nux Vomica
(Poison nut, vomiting nut)

In health the person needing *Nux vomica* will be very involved with her work. She has a lively, enquiring, inventive mind, is full of ideas and is willing to make the effort to carry them out. She will drive herself to achieve perfection and will want others to work as hard and be as quick on the uptake as she is. Where she is opposed, contradicted or otherwise held up she will be impatient, irritable, angry, even violent; she is extremely sensitive to obstacles.

She is constantly trying to push herself beyond what her system can cope with. She wants to do more than she can, both emotionally and physically. She can put herself in the position of being over-promoted and then being unable to do all she wants to.

She is a perfectionist and tends to be orderly and methodical, though not in the fussy way of *Arsenicum*. She appears to be very self-confident and decisive, never talks about worries or doubts and acts quickly to resolve tension, sometimes too impulsively.

However, there is often a driven feeling behind all this. For all the obvious pleasure and enjoyment she derives from a busy and active life, there is a sense that the woman cannot choose. Sometimes the drive behind this personality pattern is a profound need for admiration and approval. She needs to be successful and is very competitive. She can never be satisfied with herself; failure is seen as humiliation. Her pride is easily wounded.

She experiences extraordinary anxiety about many things: work, the future, financial security, physical security, health. She will not be paralysed by these anxieties or even talk about them but will try to sort them out, overcome them. For instance, an anxiety about money will be dealt with by working harder, working out a method of earning more; an anxiety about health will be resolved by going to the doctor for a check or starting on a fitness programme.

She cannot relax without help: she is the kind of person who will use drugs and stimulants to relax or to keep going. She will begin by having a mild tranquillizer or a drink in the evening and may find herself caught in a spiral of addiction. She may eat too much, drink too much alcohol and coffee, work too hard, stay up too late, smoke too much. She may drive herself into the ground with overwork and overuse of stimulants. When exhausted she can become very depressed and even suicidal; she will be unable to sleep or will wake early in the morning (3 a.m.) thinking about what she has to do or planning what she might do, never satisfied.

Underneath all this she is also emotional and sensitive, easily hurt. She is as quick with her sympathy and kindness as she is with her irritability and anger. She is concerned for the health of others but not for herself.

Her nervous system becomes oversensitive: she is disturbed by light and noise: very small noises disturb her, even the noise of someone eating an apple can set her teeth on edge. She is very sensitive to smells. Allergic reactions to various scents and pollens may develop. Nervous twitchy spasmodic movements are common in all parts of the body. She is jumpy.

This picture of nervous system sensitivity, general irritability and quick anger also often appears as a result of abuse of drugs and alcohol in a person who has not previously been inclined to such symptoms.

Physically the person who needs *Nux vomica* is likely to be very chilly. She hates the cold and catches cold easily, especially if exposed to draughts or chilled. She hates dry windy weather and is much better if she can be warm and completely covered up when ill.

Many of her complaints are digestive; she is what used to be called 'bilious': everything affects her stomach. She craves, eats and is aggravated by fatty foods, spicy food, sour food, alcohol, coffee and condiments, and dislikes bread and meat. She is as intolerant of foods as of people and vomiting is frequent, or nausea with inability to vomit. She is always better for vomiting, for getting things out. Food is not properly digested or evacuated because of the spasmodic behaviour of the stomach. Constipation is frequent with ineffectual urging, once more she 'wants to but can't.' It often alternates with diarrhoea, especially diarrhoea from juicy fruit. She can become averse to food altogether and become anorexic.

Headaches are usually associated with eating or drinking unwisely or overwork. A *Nux vomica* headache is like a hangover and is better for lying down and resting, wrapping up warmly.

Spasm, interrupted action, runs through the picture. Colds are characteristically blocked up and stuffy with a dry tickly spasmodic cough. Eyes will be sensitive to light. Breathing is spasmodic when the sufferer has a cold, asthma, hay fever, allergic rhinitis. There is spasmodic sneezing: a lot of it, the sufferer can sneeze for a long time on waking; hiccoughs are common.

The menstrual cycle is the focus for many *Nux* problems: the sufferer is irritable before periods, often to the point of real anger and violence; during them she has severe cramping and spasmodic pain, low back pain and heavy bleeding; she can also have bleeding between them. They can often be irregular, spasmodic. Cystitis can be a recurring problem: the condition fits the general picture of *Nux* very well with its urgent but ineffectual desire to urinate. She will suffer from nausea and piles during pregnancy; also possibly from back pain due to muscle spasm, low back pain or lumbago. In the menopause there may be hot flushes due to the spasmodic blood supply.

Better: sleep, nap, heat, warmth, evening, wet applications, firm pressure.

Worse: morning on waking, after meals, coffee, alcohol, cold, cold dry weather, cold dry winds, (especially east), spices, drugs, overwork, anger, sedentary life, noise, 3-4 a.m., loss of sleep.

Nux vomica is characterized by **intensity**. Everything is overdone.

The person who needs it **works very hard, eats** and **drinks too much,** uses too much **alcohol** and **stimulants,** is a **critical** and **self-critical perfectionist** who cannot achieve all she wants. She can become **irritable** and **angry,** especially when **contradicted** or opposed. She is **oversensitive** physically and emotionally. She is extremely **chilly.** Her digestive system is chronically disturbed: she is **bilious** and **constipated, craves spicy foods. Spasmodic activity** and **movements** are characteristic.

This used to be thought of primarily as a man's remedy and the more unbridled expressions of the temperament will still be seen more commonly in men. However, this should not blind us to the extraordinary usefulness of the remedy for women, even though the symptoms may appear to be milder. It may be indicated in addiction, allergies to food or pollens, anorexia, anxiety, backache, colds, colic, constipation, hay fever, headache, hiccoughs, indigestion, irritable bowel syndrome, morning sickness, piles, ulcers.

Phosphorus

The woman who needs *Phosphorus* is in health sociable, charming, affectionate, entertaining and easily emotional. She is outgoing, always looking for a response from and interaction with other people. She likes to please and is generous, open and helpful by nature. However, she may become quite withdrawn if her affection and openness is not returned; she needs attention and reassurance, especially through physical, even sexual, contact. She has a high sex drive and can become anxious in later life, fearing that she will become less attractive.

She is very imaginative and artistic in temperament, feels things strongly, is very sensitive to emotional atmospheres. She can be over-sympathetic, identifying with the feelings, thoughts and interests of others to such an extent as to lose any sense of her separate identity. This blurring of 'boundaries' is reflected also in her relationship with the spirit world, which may seem as real to her as everyday life. She may take for granted the presence of ghosts or spirits, have prophetic dreams, 'know' when those she loves are ill or distressed. The sensitivity is also physical: she is sensitive to smells, to light, to changes in temperature or weather, to electrical changes in atmosphere, to noises.

She can be very up and down emotionally, giving way to tantrums or outbursts of rage which are quickly over. Alternation between excitement and depression, between high energy and collapse is highly characteristic, though it is much less intense than in *Lachesis*. She is easily enthusiastic and interested in many things, then becomes easily bored or loses energy. She is an intuitive thinker with a short attention span, moving quickly from one interest and one person to another, not liking to be limited or trapped in one place. This may lead to her being unable to finish things or really to get to grips with anything.

Her nervous system is delicate and impressionable; she is easily startled and full of fears and anxieties. She is terrified of what may happen in the future, has deep fears of being alone, especially in the dark at night when her imagination is heightened; she is anxious about disease and death. She is terrified of thunderstorms. She has vivid dreams and nightmares.

She is prone to nervous exhaustion and can be quite weak and delicate physically, despite the vitality of her nature. She gets totally exhausted and unable to make any kind of effort. She can become irritable and apathetic and doesn't want to think, talk or work. She is easily debilitated by illness and needs sympathy and company.

She is also debilitated by loss of blood. Bleeding is a prominent feature of the remedy, often to the extent of causing anaemia. Cuts, gums and noses bleed easily; ulcers and piles bleed; discharges tend to be blood-streaked; she bruises easily. There's very heavy menstrual bleeding, with bright red clotted blood, to the point of haemorrhage sometimes.

Her circulation is very variable: though generally chilly she can be hot and cold in parts and suffers from burning sensations in particular spots. She gets hot flushes within and without the menopause. Her feet, hands and knees can be icy cold, especially at night. Her circulation is noticeably affected by emotion, she easily gets palpitations and feelings of faintness and suffocation. Palpitations are worse lying on the left side and she only sleeps on the right side.

She presents a low blood sugar picture, frequently feeling faint and dizzy when hungry and craving sweet things. She is hungry before going to bed, wakes at 3 a.m. hungry, is hungry at breakfast time, hungry at 11 a.m. She gets a characteristic 'gone', empty, weak sensation which is not better for eating. She eats a lot and yet stays thin, since she metabolizes food very quickly. She gets a headache when hungry (better for cold compresses).

She is exceptionally thirsty and always for cold or iced drinks, especially milk; she craves cold food too. Hot food and drinks can make her feel sick and even cold food and drinks can bring on this feeling by the time they have warmed up in the stomach.

She craves fat, salt, spicy things, meat, cold milk, ice cream. She dislikes beer, meat, tea, boiled milk and oysters. She can crave or loathe fish and fizzy drinks.

Burning pains in the stomach associated with the hungry faint sensation are characteristic. The pains are worse for heat and better for cold food and drink. She can have nausea which is worse for putting hands in cold water and for drinking water. She has a peculiar kind of constipation with long slender hard dry stools. She can also suffer from profuse and exhausting diarrhoea.

The remedy is very well indicated where chest and lungs are affected. Colds start in the head and move quickly to the chest, usually accompanied by a sore throat, with a raw burning sensation. The throat is very sensitive to touch and cold air, hoarseness and loss of voice is common and worse towards the evening. A hard dry tickly cough develops which is worse when the person first lies down, worse lying on the left side, moving from warm to cold or from cold to warm; better sitting up.

Pains are usually burning pains, wherever they are. Symptoms tend to be left-sided.

Better: company, cold drinks, sleep, heat (except head and stomach), eating, rubbing, being touched, fresh air, lying on right side.

Worse: cold, thunderstorms, lightning, lying on left side, twilight and dark, heights, before eating, change of weather, wind, physical or mental exertion, hot meals and drinks, lying on painful side.

The picture of *Phosphorus* is of a person who can be **restless** and **excitable, weak** and **exhausted.** The woman who needs it will be extremely nervous, **anxious** and **fearful** especially in the **dark,** about **health, thunderstorms.** She **craves company,** is usually **sympathetic** but an extreme **indifference** can set in. She is **affectionate, interested in sex.** She has an **active mind** and **imagination.** She is **chilly, worse** for **cold, better** for **heat.** Craves **salt, spicy foods** and **ice cream. Burning pains, easy bleeding** and an **empty hungry sensation** not better for eating are characteristic. Symptoms tend to be **left-sided.**

If the general symptoms agree it may be strongly indicated in heavy bleeding, bronchitis, chesty colds, diabetes, kidney problems, mastitis, morning sickness, nose bleeds, palpitations, sore throats.

Phytolacca decandra
(Pokeroot)

The emotional symptoms of this remedy are not yet very clear, but there is a certain gloomy indifference to people and things along with an expectation of imminent death; also some irritability.

Pains come and go suddenly and move around rapidly from one place to another; they shoot upwards. There is marked tiredness and weakness: the sufferer is worn out and always wanting to lie down. She aches all over and feels bruised, sore and battered. The glands are hard, painful and swollen. She is generally chilly and complaints tend to be right-sided.

The throat is often affected: it is sore with rawness, roughness, stiff neck muscles and painful tonsils. Pain shoots into the ears especially when swallowing; it is worse for hot drinks and worse on the right side. Patient feels she has a foreign object in her throat which hurts when she sticks out her tongue. Swallowing may become impossible. Breath smells.

The breasts may be sore and lumpy before and during menstrual periods with stony hard painful nodules, better for pressure of hand. There is pain in the breast when nursing. Milk is apt to coagulate and hang in strings from the nipples. It is useful in acute mastitis: breast is stony, hard, painful and tender. Breast abscesses are possible. Helpful for sore and cracked nipples when baby is feeding. Pain radiates all over the body. Periods are frequent, heavy and painful with membranous blood.

There are sensations of stiffness and bruising all over the body. Pains are worse for cold wet weather and better for warm dry weather. Movement is painful: there is an urge to move but the sufferer is afraid to do so. Joints become swollen, hard, tender and intensely hot. Shooting pains, like electric shocks, come and go suddenly, move around, upwards. Sciatic pain on right side.

Better: dry weather, lying on left side, when warm.

Worse: cold, especially damp cold, thundery weather, rain, weather changes, motion, menstruation, night, lying on right side.

Phytolacca is **sore and bruised** and particularly affects the **throat, breasts** and **joints.** Pains which **shoot** from place to place, and a **stony hardness** are characteristic.

It may be thought of in the following conditions: mastitis, mumps, muscle and joint pain, cracked nipples, sciatica, sore throat, teething, tonsillitis.

Pulsatilla (Wind flower)

In *Pulsatilla* there is a state of changeableness and instability. The sufferer's circulation is unstable: feelings of being hot or cold alternately, she is sometimes hot and cold in different parts of her body; she can be chilly in a warm room yet cannot bear warm stuffy atmospheres and has to have fresh air. She gets too hot in bed then gets too cold; she has cold fingers with white ends. All systems (especially digestive and menstrual) are easily disturbed by many things: temperature, climate, food for example. Symptoms in general are variable: no two attacks of anything are alike. Pains are also variable. They appear suddenly and go away gradually (or the reverse). They shift around the body.

The temperament reflects the physical state. The person is easy-going, shy, gentle and malleable in temperament, yielding. She is likely to be emotional, tearful, changeable: happy and sad in turn. She cries easily and is generally better for crying, though can become quite depressed if alone and unsupported. She is friendly and likes the company of others. If she is ill she seeks reassurance and is better for consolation and company, and being in her own home with friends, family and familiar things. The remedy is often indicated in clingy, tearful children who cannot bear mother to be out of sight, in school phobia etc. The *Pulsatilla* woman is easily affected and changed, is easily pushed around by others, takes on the opinions of others in order to get the approval she needs, is indecisive in her own right.

Conversely, there is a congested state: catarrh is marked and there is congestion of blood in the veins. There is a tendency to frequent catarrhal colds, headaches, blocked ears (glue ear) as well as to catarrhal discharges in the genital area. Discharges are yellow, yellowy-green, creamy. The remedy has a great affinity to the veins: it comes into play at the menopause and is indicated in the hot flushes, varicose veins and piles which may manifest then or during pregnancy.

Temperamentally, the woman has a fragile sense of self-esteem which makes her touchy and easily hurt, though not aggressive or violent. She needs a lot of open affection and reassurance, is very sensitive to criticism. She is timid and has many fears: of being alone, of the dark, of ghosts, of crowds, of open spaces, of going insane. She can develop strange preoccupations and convictions, for instance that certain foods should not be eaten, that the opposite sex is dangerous; or religious ideas which may reach the stage of obsession.

She has a lot of headaches, is inclined to have them with any complaint, especially if it is digestive or to do with menstruation. The eyes and ears are often affected. The eyes are watery and there is a tendency to styes, conjunctivitis and even corneal ulceration. The ears join in the general catarrhal condition and there is often deafness and earache after a cold: there can be a thick creamy pussy discharge.

Catarrhal colds are characteristic, with the nose blocked in a warm room and at night; the cough is dry and tickly at night. Both are freer in day and outdoors. Long-lasting catarrhal states with thick yellowish or green bland discharge. Very dry sore throat without thirst. Hay fever.

Digestion is difficult and slow with heartburn, bloatedness, belching. The sufferer craves cool food and juicy fruit, lemon drinks. She also craves pastries, fat, rich foods and ice cream, all of which disagree with her. She dislikes meat, especially pork, milk, butter. Nausea and vomiting are frequent, from emotional upset. Piles are painful and itchy, worse from warmth of bed.

Menstruation is characteristically late to start in young girls and irregular once started, often with pain, nausea and fainting. Amenorrhoea (absence of periods) is common: periods stop for the slightest reason and tend to be irregular, delayed, changeable, scanty. Premenstrually weepy, touchy and irritable. Also breasts are painful before and during periods (can have cysts). There may be milk in breasts outside pregnancy. Nausea, vomiting, diarrhoea, back pain and headache also common before or during periods. During period loss of appetite, cutting tearing pains in lower abdomen and back. In later life periods tend to continue to be irregular: flow can be either scanty or profuse, often with clots. There is a tendency to cervical erosion and prolapse. Various uterine disorders associated with thick, yellowy-green, creamy, non-irritating discharges. There is a tendency to leucorrhoea and thrush. Thrush has yellow or milky creamy discharge, either bland or irritating. Well indicated for vaginitis during pregnancy and in girls at puberty. Watery cloudy discharge which causes smarting and soreness worse before and after periods and when lying down. Cystitis with significant smarting and burning. It is highly indicated in stress incontinence, especially when sneezing or lying down.

It is useful in disorders of pregnancy with uterine inertia, feeble labour pains, abnormal presentation.

Pale complexion, inclined to be anaemic. Easily feels faint, headachy, dizzy, nauseous. Palpitation and hot flushes accompany anxiety states or emotional upset and may occur after a heavy meal. Tendency to put on weight and retain fluid. Generally thirstless (marked in acute cases).

Better: fresh open air, cold dry air, cold food, cool applications, pressure, lying on the painful part, gentle movement, sympathy, consolation, pregnancy.

Worse: heat and stuffy rooms, humidity, too many clothes or bed clothes, rest, lying on left side, evening, eating rich or fatty foods.

Pulsatilla is **clingy, changeable, sensitive, tearful, emotional, irritable, timid, chilly** but **worse** for **warm rooms, better** for **company, thirstless.**

It may be thought of in the following conditions: breech presentation, children's illnesses, stuffy colds, cystitis, earache, indigestion, measles, mumps, palpitations, period pains, piles, PMS, rheumatism, varicose veins.

Rhus tox
(Poison ivy or poison oak)

Extreme restlessness is both a psychological and a physical characteristic of this remedy. The patient cannot get comfortable, and needs to keep moving. She suffers from painful stiffness of muscles and joints which is worse on first movement and better for slow continued motion. She is much worse after rest. Worse with tiredness, over-exertion. The pains are characteristically shooting and tearing and accompanied by stiffness. Almost all symptoms are worse for cold damp weather or conditions, better in hot dry weather or conditions: headache, skin, rheumatism.

She suffers from restless anxiety and worry about all sorts of things: the future, the family, business. She can be nervous and irritable with sadness and thoughts of suicide: weary of life. She may burst into tears for no particular reason. The anxiety is worse in bed at night when she has to be still, especially after midnight when her mind dwells on unpleasant past events; she is better for walking in the fresh air. She has a great anxiety and fear of being poisoned, even by medicines.

Small blister-like eruptions appear on the skin: they are about the size of a pinhead and filled with a transparent liquid. The skin is red, itchy, burning and swollen, especially at night or if hot. It is relieved by hot compresses or showers, not by scratching.

In illness the tongue is dry and sore, coated white or brown and has the strange, rare and peculiar symptom (see page 36) of a red triangular tip.

Characteristically the sufferer has an unquenchable thirst for cold drinks, especially at night. Desire for cold milk and sweets; dislike of meat and bread.

Better: movement, changing position; warm dry bed, weather, clothes; hot drinks, hot applications.

Worse: getting wet, change of weather to cold/damp, autumn, getting chilled, cold cloudy foggy wet weather, swimming in cold water; cold drinks, cold food, damp, draughts; first movement, rest, sitting, lying down, lying on right side; evening especially around 7 p.m., night, especially second half.

The characteristic symptoms of *Rhus tox* are **anxiety** and **restlessness, painful stiffness worse on first beginning to move, better for slow continued movement** but worse again if continues too long and gets overtired, **worse** for **over-exertion**. Almost all symptoms are **worse** for **cold damp**.

The remedy may be indicated in gout, herpes, jaw pain, low fevers (flu, typhoid, rheumatic) mumps, muscle and joint pain, sciatica.

Sepia
(Cuttlefish ink)

Sepia is derived from the inky protective cloud put out as a disguise by the cuttlefish, a slightly more advanced mollusc than the oyster from which *Calc carb* is derived. Something of the sense of the remedy may be picked up by thinking of one of those old sepia photographs with their uniform brown tinge and suggestion of life having been suspended while everyone smiles into the camera. *Sepia* is great at smiling into the camera and getting on with things.

In health *Sepia* is a vital, hard-working woman who will take on anything. While she is fit enough to work hard she has abundant energy, is full of life, intelligent, assertive, direct. She is highly competent, at work or in running a family, and sees no reason why she should apologize for that. She is deeply emotional but is not ruled by her emotions, as is *Pulsatilla*, for example: she has a strong mind and will.

However, when the adrenalin runs out, and exhaustion sets in, the woman who needs *Sepia* becomes quite worn out and an almost opposite state is seen: a burned-out, drooping, depleted state. She will sag and droop mentally and physically. If she can counter the stagnation by activity, she will be able to pick up: she is always better for vigorous exercise, dancing or fast walking and worse for rest, even when exhausted. However, when she gets too weary to exercise then she is completely overcome by the exhaustion.

Her mood ranges from weepy and irritable to profound depression. She can be anxious and agitated, wanting to scream, run away from home, leave the family. Nobody can help: she cries when asked questions and is irritable if consoled or sympathized with. She is irritable about everything: small noises, being contradicted. This can change to a state of enormous indifference: she does not care about anything, about her family or loved ones especially, her work, what she looks like, what her house looks like. She 'can't be bothered', is worn out; she sits and does nothing: nothing has any meaning; she becomes completely uninterested in sex.

Many of the difficulties in the *Sepia* remedy picture are caused by or appear in conjunction with rather complicated and often serious gynaecological problems. It is an important remedy in hormonal imbalance. Irritability or despair is marked before periods. Dryness of the vagina is a frequent complication and may contribute to the development of an aversion to sexual activity; she tends to leucorrhoea and genital infections which bring her down. Heavy periods are a feature of the remedy. There is a general pelvic weakness: she has poor muscle tone and feels as if there is something heavy inside dragging her down. She might have to sit with her legs crossed because of a sensation that the womb will fall out. Nausea accompanies many gynaecological problems, and the remedy is superb in morning sickness.

The veins take part in the general lack of tone: there are varicose veins and piles, strong venous congestion.

The circulation is very strongly affected. The woman is very chilly, feels the cold easily. A peculiar feature is that sometimes the upper and lower limbs are different temperatures. She catches cold easily, especially after getting wet. She sweats easily and profusely, with a sour smell. She has frequent feelings as if hot flushes were occurring but there is little actual redness; there is a lot of sweating and fainting.

It is like *Nux vomica* and *Lycopodium* in being a liverish sort of remedy. You can tell that the liver is not working fully because of a slight yellowness of eyes and skin; whitish stools, offensive gases from the bowels and red sediment in the urine.

The sufferer will be bloated and constipated and feel full after only a small amount of food: more often has a 'gone', empty feeling, however. She often complains of a sensation of a ball or lump in the throat, abdomen, rectum or womb. She craves vinegar, pickles, acidy, spicy, bitter or highly seasoned foods. Dislikes meat, especially fat on meat, milk. She may develop such an aversion to food that she cannot stand its smell: the smell may cause intense nausea. She may have a gnawing sensation of emptiness in the stomach or abdomen that food does not satisfy.

Better: eating, vigorous exercise, running, fast walking, dancing, elevating the legs.

Worse: before/during/after menstrual period, cold, fasting, getting wet, rest, sweating, touch, mental exertion, kneeling, storm brewing, left side, 4-6 p.m., morning.

Sepia is a remedy for a woman who is highly **active** when well and when ill is **irritable, exhausted, indifferent** to everything and everybody, **averse** to **sex**. However she is **better** for **vigorous exercise** and **dancing**. She is **chilly** but subject to **hot flushes**.

This remedy may be indicated in problems of backache and rheumatism, constipation, depression, digestive problems, M.E., menopause, menstruation, morning sickness, piles, prolapse, varicose veins.

Silica

In *Silica* what is remarkable is the general low level of energy, both physical and mental. Some people even describe this as inertia. There is a general lack of response to both life and illness. They are always weak and tired and wanting to lie down: delicate children with little resistance.

A person needing *Silica* is likely to appear quite weak-looking and thin (though she need not be). Food is not assimilated properly and there is consequent undernourishment and debility. Bones do not form well. They may have weak ankles and be slow learning to walk, slow teething; the fontanelles close slowly. It's appropriate to the kind of children who fail to thrive. There's a demineralized state, a state almost of malnutrition.

The subject is always cold, and easily gets chilled; is very sensitive to draughts and a cold wind. She has icy-cold hands and feet and wears a hat in summer. She catches cold very easily, and may have glandular problems and earaches.

The nervous system is oversensitive: people who need *Silica* are oversensitive to small noises, to pain, to insult too. Perhaps because of this they are timid, fearful and anxious. They are particularly fearful of undertaking anything, for fear they will fail. They fear appearing in public because of this. However, if they do decide to undertake something, they will work very hard and conscientiously and do it very well. They can develop quite a lot of quiet perseverance and confidence in themselves providing they keep out of situations which challenge them too much. In fact they are prone to overwork, they are so conscientious. They can be extremely obstinate and self-willed and can become quite obsessional. Their aim in life never wavers and they will work hard to achieve it. They can also go the other way and suffer from lack of concentration. They are quick-minded.

The remedy has a state of suppuration, like *Hepar sulph*, but the process is much slower in *Silica*. There are a lot of slow-maturing abscesses. Patients sweat profusely especially at night and on back of head and neck (like *Calc carb*, though not so profusely) and have smelly sweaty feet (socks rot) and poor circulation. Nails have white spots and break easily. Skin is dry with cracks at corners of mouth. There is a characteristic constipation where the stool slips back as it is about to emerge, 'shy stool'.

Better: summer, warmth and being wrapped up warmly, especially the head, hot applications.

Worse: morning, cold damp, draughts, cold wind, milk, new moon, pressure, periods, vaccinations.

Silica is **chilly, undernourished, timid and anxious** yet **obstinate** and even **obsessional. Suppuration** is strong.

It may be indicated in boils, bronchitis, constipation, festering cuts, ear infections, eczema, eye infections, glandular fever, M.E., tonsillitis.

Staphysagria
(Stavesacre, Larkspur, Delphinium)

The strongest characteristic of *Staphysagria* lies in the nature of its response to emotional injury. It has been called the *Arnica* of the psyche. A person needing *Staphysagria* cannot express feelings when hurt and pretends that nothing has happened. It will be needed in any condition resulting from failure to express feelings of anger, indignation, humiliation, grief, rejection.

Sometimes the failure to express appropriate feelings arises because of an unequal situation: for instance being criticized or judged by a boss or a husband; sometimes the inability becomes chronic, arising from a life-long adaptation, begun in childhood, when expression of feelings in face of the parents was too dangerous.

If it is a life-long adaptation, it is possible that the woman will be unconscious of it and will genuinely believe herself to be as mild and agreeable as she appears to others. In a more acute state the temporarily suppressed feelings may erupt in either a physical complaint such as eczema or colicky stomach ache, or in a fit of displaced anger, when the sufferer may throw or break things.

However well it is suppressed, the true state may be revealed by the woman's touchiness and oversensitivity to the slightest thing; she easily feels she is being got at. She is easily irritated and excitable. She may develop physical symptoms rather than express feelings: she feels exhausted and shaky, trembles inside. She is upset when people are rude to her. The key symptom is 'reserved displeasure'.

This remedy is well indicated where a woman has been bullied or abused and humiliated in some way, particularly where she has not apparently responded angrily. It is a remedy for any situation where the subject has been unable for whatever reason to respond directly to some kind of injustice, vexation, humiliation, contempt or emotional rejection.

It is often indicated in the effects of sexual abuse, for instance where intellectual and psychological development has been interrupted, or there is distortion of the body image in anorexia. Obsessional sexual ideas which are extremely disturbing may develop.

There are several physical characteristics of the remedy, sometimes arising from suppressed emotion or accompanying the expression of emotion. So for example, coughs, headaches, stomach aches, cystitis, exhaustion all resulting from the suppression of anger or accompanying its delayed expression.

It is also an important remedy for the effects of physical injuries, lacerations, especially where these are accompanied by feelings of humiliation and anger. It is well indicated after surgical operations, especially in the sexual, genital area: episiotomy or hysterectomy, for example, and in cystitis after intercourse. It is important after any experience perceived as sexual assault.

There are some important characteristic physical features, for example a proneness to styes. Blackened crumbling teeth are also part of the remedy picture; it can also have exquisitely painful toothache. A strange, rare and peculiar symptom (see page 36) is that there is a sensation of stitches in the ear on swallowing. It is well indicated in tonsillitis and has glandular affections.

Better: warmth, rest, eating.

Worse: exertion, fasting, tobacco, touch, mental exertion, disappointment, sexual excess.

Staphysagria is characterized by **suppressed indignation** and **resentment,** and pent-up **anger. Sensitivity** to **pain** is marked and sufferers are **worse** for **touch.**

It may be indicated in anger, anorexia, colic, cystitis, headache, lacerated wounds, muscle and joint pains, resentment, styes, effects of sexual abuse, rape, effects of surgical operation, tonsillitis.

Sulphur

Some people who need *Sulphur* might be very easy to spot initially. They look a little eccentric, wearing old or unfashionable casual clothes, apparently indifferent to their personal appearance. At one end of the spectrum they can be dirty and even smelly, since they have a strong dislike of washing; they smell bad but are usually unaware of it. They may also look very hot: they're usually warm-blooded and uncomfortable in a warm room. They crave fresh air.

They may look a little red in the face and may have red edges to eyelids or mouth (all orifices may have red edges). They don't like standing up straight and will lean against things, will always be wanting to sit or even lie down. If they sit they will slide down in the chair.

Just as they don't dress conventionally, so they won't behave conventionally either. They won't be polite if they don't want to be, not that they will be downright rude but just that they are very self-absorbed and tend to talk a lot about whatever is interesting them at the time: if that doesn't interest others they still carry on. You can feel very alone with a *Sulphur*.

They are the kind of people who say that their thermostat has broken. The circulation is disturbed. They overheat easily, or the blood flows unevenly: head may be hot and feet cold. Feet get very hot in bed at night and have to be stuck out of the bedclothes. When the weather changes from cold to warm they are uncomfortable. They dislike extreme cold, though. Their blood vessels feel too full and there will be sensations of burning, heat, inflammation and itchy eruptions.

They sweat profusely (often sour and smelly) and feel worse while sweating; worse for menopausal hot flushes. Discharges are hot, smelly and burning. Always feel tired, cannot go to sleep early: sleep does not refresh. They are markedly worse for exertion and therefore avoid it and are often called lazy. They sleep in in the mornings.

The skin is dry, harsh and rough with a tendency to pussy spots which are difficult to heal. It is dry, hot and very itchy at night in bed. The itchiness can be relieved by scratching until the skin bleeds, but then it is sore and water aggravates it so it is much worse for washing.

They are frequently hungry, ravenously so, and can't eat enough to satisfy their appetite: they get indigestion after eating. Everything is worse around 11 a.m., they have a 'gone' sensation in the stomach which is worse for missing meals. They get indigestion after eating. They tend to like spicy foods, sweets, fat and alcohol and to dislike meat and milk (they may also dislike or be aggravated by sweets and fats.) Very thirsty for large quantities. Diarrhoea at 5 a.m. drives them from bed.

Untidiness is a feature. They live in a mess, physically and mentally. They start things and don't finish them. They never put things away and they never throw things away either, they collect and hoard things. Their minds are like huge attics full of half-finished projects, ideas, schemes. They always have something to tell, some curious facts. They can't finish projects because they collect too much information and are unable to select or refine it. They are very curious but undisciplined. They are interested in ideas, philosophies, questions impossible to answer. It is very difficult for them to ground ideas. They are very intuitive, full of hunches, seeing infinite possibilities in a situation, but rarely realizing them in practical terms.

They are normally too introspective and self-concerned to be aggressive to people: they ignore others rather than attack, but they are easily offended and can be critical, irritable and quarrelsome if challenged. They dislike people who offend them and can become quite morose and suspicious.

All this is a cover, of course, for anxiety and low self-esteem. Although they can be haughty and egotistical, they also have a melancholy anxious side to them. They totter between the two modes. They can become quite seriously anxious and depressed, to the point of wanting to die, and with the depression comes an impatience, irritability and moroseness which doesn't endear them to those who try to help. Weeping is marked especially during periods and during the menopause.

They are anxious quite a lot of the time, especially in bed and about the future. They can become anxious about a whole range of moral and religious questions, the possibility of catching diseases. There can in illness be a quite fussy, picky aspect to them reminiscent of *Arsenicum*. In the end they can become so self-absorbed and indifferent to others that they become separate from other people and live in a world of their own. This makes them unhappy because, despite appearances, they need confirmation from others: they feel unrecognized and unappreciated and don't understand how it happened.

Better: sweating, motion, dry weather, fresh air, lying on the right side.

Worse: standing still, heat of bed, water, morning 11 a.m., after sleeping, bathing, change of weather to warm, draughts, exertion, fasting, heat, stuffy rooms, lying on the left side.

Sulphur is one of the major remedies in homoeopathy. It is characterized by its **heat, redness, burning** and **itching. Burning pains** and **discharges** and **smelliness** are marked. They are **worse at 11 a.m., worse** for **warmth, better** in **open air,** averse to and **worse** for **washing. Untidy** and incapable of completing things they are **discontented** and **eccentric.** They are **curious** and **introspective.** They can be **depressed** and **irritable.**

It may be indicated in alcoholism, anxiety, asthma, backache, bulimia, clearing up lingering complaints, depression, diarrhoea, eczema, glandular fever, indigestion, itchy skin, menopausal complaints, M.E., piles, rheumatism.

Appendix One

FURTHER READING

Martin L Budd, *Low Blood Sugar*, Thorsons 1984.

Miranda Castro, *The Complete Homoeopathy Handbook: A Guide to Everyday Health Care*, Macmillan 1990.

Leon Chaitow, *Vaccination and Immunisation: Dangers, Delusions and Alternatives*, C W Daniel 1987.

Stephen Cummings and Dana Ullmann, *Everybody's Guide to Homoeopathic Medicines: Taking Care of Yourself and Your Family with Safe and Effective Remedies*, Gollancz 1986.

Doris Grant and Jean Joice, *Food Combining for Health*, Thorsons 1984.

Christopher Hammond, *How to Use Homoeopathy*, Element Books 1991.

Rima Handley, *A Homeopathic Love Story*, North Atlantic Books 1990.

Mary Laver and Margaret Smith, *Diet for Life*, Pan 1981. (An adaptation of the Dong Diet.)

Felicity Lee, *Vaccination, A Difficult Decision*, a leaflet published by the Society of Homoeopaths, September 1991.

Jackie Le Tissier, *Food Combining for Vegetarians*, Thorsons 1992.

Andrew Lockie, *The Family Guide to Homeopathy: The Safe Form of Medicine for the Future*, Hamish Hamilton 1990.

Randall Neustaedter, *The Immunization Decision: A Guide for Parents*, North Atlantic Books 1990.

Angela Phillips and Jill Rakusen, eds., *The New Our Bodies Ourselves*, Penguin 1989.

Dana Ullmann, *Homeopathy, Medicine for the 21st Century*, North Atlantic Books 1988.

Michael Weiner and Kathleen Goss, *The Complete Book of Homoeopathy*, Bantam 1982.

Appendix Two

———

USEFUL ADDRESSES

The Society of Homoeopaths
2 Artizan Road
Northampton
NN1 4HU

British Homoeopathic Association
27a Devonshire Street
London
W1N 1RJ

The Hahnemann Society
Humane Education Centre
Avenue Lodge
Bounds Green Road
London
NE22 4EU

Homoeopathic Development
Foundation Ltd.
Harcourt House
19a Cavendish Square
London
W1M 9AD

Council for Complementary and
Alternative Medicine
Suite 1, 19a Cavendish Square
London
W1M 9AD

Homoeopathic Hospitals

The Royal Homoeopathic Hospital
Great Ormond Street
London
WC1N 3HR

Glasgow Homoeopathic Hospital
100 Great Western Road
Glasgow
G12 0RN

Bristol Homoeopathic Hospital
Cotham Road
Cotham, Bristol
BS6 6UJ

Tunbridge Wells Homoeopathic
Hospital
Church Road
Tunbridge Wells
Kent
TN1 1JU

Department of Homoeopathic
Medicine
Mossley Hill Hospital
Park Avenue
Liverpool
L18 8BU

Homoeopathic Pharmacies and Suppliers

Ainsworths
38 New Cavendish Street
London
W1M 7LH

Galen Pharmacy
1 South Street
Dorchester
Dorset
DT1 1DE

Helios
92 Camden Road
Tunbridge Wells
Kent
TN1 2QP

Nelson's Pharmacies Limited
73 Duke Street
London
W1M 6BY

Weleda UK Limited
Heanor Road
Ilkeston, Derbyshire
DE7 8DR

Boxes and bottles for storing remedies can be obtained from:
The Homoeopathic Supply Company
4 Nelson Road
Sherringham
Norfolk
NR26 8BU

USA

Homeopathic Academy of
Naturopathic Physicians
11231 SE Market Street
Portland
Oregon 92716

North American Society of
Homeopaths
Valerie O'Hanlan
4712 Aldrich Avenue
Minneapolis
MN 55409

New Zealand

New Zealand Institute of Classical
Homeopathy
Gwyneth Gibson
24 Westhaven Drive
Tawa, Wellington

South Africa

Joyce Bagnall
c/o AG Bagnall
PO Box 3179
Durban 400
Natal

Australia

Society of Classical Homeopathy
2nd Floor, Paxton House
90 Pitt Street
Sydney 2000

Canada

Murray Feldman
Vancouver Centre for Homeopathy
2246 Spruce Street
Vancouver, BC
V6H 2P3

Appendix Three

TRAINING

If you wish to undertake training to practise homoeopathic medicine, the following courses are available:

The College of Homoeopathy
Regent's College
Inner Circle
London
NW1 4NS

The Northern College of
Homeopathic Medicine
Swinburne House
Swinburne Street
Gateshead
Tyne and Wear
NE8 1AX

The London College of Classical
Homoeopathy
Morley College
61 Westminster Bridge Road
London
SE1 7HT

The School of Homoeopathy
Yondercott House
Uffculme
Devon
EX15 3DR

The British School of Homoeopathy
23 Sarum Avenue
Melksham
Wiltshire
SN12 6BN

The College of Classical
Homoeopathy
Othergates Clinic
45 Barringon Street
Tiverton
Devon
EX16 6QP

The North West College of
Homoeopathy
23 Wilbraham Road
Fallowfield
Manchester
M14 6FB

Appendix Four: Materia Medica

Abbreviated Name	Remedy
Acon	Aconitum napellus
Apis	Apis mellifica
Agaricus	Agaricus muscarius
Arg n	Argentum nitricum
Arn	Arnica montana
Ars	Arsenicum album
Bel	Belladonna
Bry	Bryonia alba
Calc	Calcarea carbonica
Cal	Calendula
Canth	Cantharis
Carb	Carbo vegetabilis
Caul	Caulophyllum
Caust	Causticum
Cham	Chamomilla
Chin	China
Cimi	Cimicifuga
Coloc	Colocynthis
Coffea	Coffea cruda
Con	Conium maculatum
Gels	Gelsemium sempervirens
Hep	Hepar sulphuris calcareum
Hyp	Hypericum perforatum
Ign	Ignatia amara
Ipec	Ipecacuanha
Kali	Kali carbonicum

Lach	Lachesis
Lyc	Lycopodium clavatum
Merc	Mercurius solubilis
Nat m	Natrum muriaticum
Nat sulph	Natrum sulphuricum
Nux	Nux vomica
Phos	Phosphorus
Phyt	Phytolacca decandra
Puls	Pulsatilla nigricans
Rhus	Rhus toxicodendron
Rut	Ruta graveolens
Sep	Sepia
Sil	Silica
Spong	Spongia tosta
Stap	Staphysagria
Sul	Sulphur
Symp	Symphytum officinale
Urt	Urtica urens

INDEX

Including Index of Symptoms

fevers *acon, apis, ars, bell, bry, calc, chin, gels, puls, rhus*

fibroids *calc, phos, sil,* 104

flatulence *arg n, carb v, cham, chin, kali, lyc, nux, sul*

fluid retention *apis, ars, kali, nat m*

food, aggravates fat *carb v, caust, chin, nat m, puls, sep*
   fruit *bry, chin, puls*
   ices *ars, ipec, puls*
   milk *bry, calc, chin, lyc, puls, sil*
   onions *lyc, nux, puls*
   pastries *lyc, phos, puls*
   pork, veal *ipec, puls, sep*
   rich *carb v, puls, sep*
   shellfish *carb v, lyc*
   averse butter *chin, merc, puls*
   eggs *calc*
   fat *calc, chin, merc, nux, sep*
   milk *calc, phos, puls, sil, sul*
   desires alcohol *chin, lach, nux, sul*
   bread *calc, nat m*
   coal, chalk, pencils *calc*
   eggs, cheese *calc*
   fat *nux, phos, puls, sul*
   indigestible things *calc*
   lemon *bell, puls*
   milk *apis, calc, merc, rhus*
   pastries, rich foods *puls*
   sensitivity *calc, kali*
   thirst for cold drinks *acon, ars, bry, cham, merc, phos, rhus*
   thirst for large amounts *ars, bry, phos, sul*
   thirst for large amounts cold *acon, bry, nat m, sul*
   thirst little and often *ars, lyc*
   thirstless *apis, bell, chin, gel, ipec, pul*
   thirsty *ars, cham, lach, merc, phos*

food, cannot bear sight, smell or thought of *ars, sep*

food-poisoning, esp from meat *ars*
   from fish *carb v*

fright, effects of *acon, apis, caust*

gastroenteritis *acon, arg n, ars, bry, chin, nux, phos*

German measles *acon, bell, bry, puls*

glands affected *bell, calc, merc, phyt, puls, sil, stap, sul*

gout *arn, lyc, rhus, sul, tox*

grief *acon, caust, ign, lach, nat m, puls, stap,* 55 *ff*

gums affected *merc, sil*

haemorrhage *see* bleeding, heavy

hangover *nux*

hasty, hurried *arg n, hep, merc*

hay fever *apis, ars, gels, ipec, nat m, nux, puls, sul*

head injuries *arn, nat sul,* 94

headache *acon, arg n, arn, ars, bell, bry, calc, cimi, ign, lach, lyc, merc, nat m, nux, phos, puls*
   bursting, throbbing *bell, bry, gels, lach, nux*
   catarrhal *merc, nux, puls*
   with any complaints *bry, puls*
   with menstrual problems *cimi, lach, nat m, puls*

heartburn *calc, carb v, lyc, nux, puls*

heatstroke *acon, bell, glon,* 94

herpes *nat m, rhus*

hiccoughs *ign, nux*

hot flushes *acon, bell, chin, cimi, lach, nux, phos, puls, sep, sul,* 100

hyperactive *calc*

hypochondriacal *nat m, nux, puls, sep, sul*

hypoglycaemia *kali, phos*

imaginative *lach, phos*

immune system 20, 21, 38

impatient, hurried *arg n, ars, bell, hep, ign, ipec, merc, nux, sep*

impressionable *phos, puls*

impulsive *arg n, hep, ign, merc, nux, puls*

incontinence *canth, caust, gels, merc, puls, sep, sul,* 113

indecisive *ars, ign, phos, puls*

indigestion *arg n, ars, bry, cham, ign, kali, lyc, merc, nux, puls, sul*

infections suppurate *hep, lach, merc, sil*

influenza *bry, gels, nux, rhus*

insomnia 59 *see also* sleeplessness

intercourse, pain during *nat m, sepia*

introspective, introverted *ign, nat m, pul, sul*

irritable *apis, bry, cham, hep, ipec, lyc, nux, phos, phyt, rhus, sep, stap, sul*

irritable bowel syndrome *lyc, nux*

jaw pain *caust, ign, phos, phyt, rhus*

jealous *apis, lach, puls, stap*

kidneys affected *acon, apis, canth, kali, lyc, phos*

laughs at serious things *nat m*

laughs easily *bell, ign*

laughs till cries *ign*

left-sided symptoms *arg n, lach, merc, nux, phos, rhus, sep, sul*

legs restless *ars, caus, rhus*

lethargic *calc, chin, gels, nux, phos, sep, sil, sul*

leucorrhoea *merc, nat m, puls, sep*

light aggravates *acon, bell, lach, nux, phos*

loquacious *see* talkative

lumbago *see* backache

lymph nodes, swollen *calc, merc*

M.E. *puls, sep, sil, sul*

mastitis *see* breasts, sore

measles *acon, bry, puls*

memory, poor *arn, lyc, merc, nat m, sep, sul*

Ménières disease *bry, chin, nat m, sil*

meningitis *apis, bry*

menopause *acon, bell, calc, cimi, kali, lach, nat m, nux, puls, sep, sul,* 97

miscarriage *acon, cimi, ign,* 78

miscarriage, threatened *arn,* 75

moody *ign, lach, phos*

morning sickness *ars, cimi, ipec, kali, merc, nux, phos, sep,* 77

morose *arn, bry, cimi, sul*

mouth ulcers *merc*

movement aggravates *arn, bell, bry, chin, kali, nux, phyt, sil, sul*

movement ameliorates *apis, ars, kali, lyc, rhus, sep*

movement fast ameliorates *sep*

  first ameliorates *arn, rhus t*

  gentle ameliorates *puls*

  slightest aggravates *bry*

mumps *apis, calc, merc, phyt, puls, rhus*

muscle and joint pain *arn, bell, bry, calc, caust, cham, cimi, kali, lyc, merc, nux, phyt, puls, rhus, rut, sep, stap, sul,* 110–111

nails break easily *sil*

nausea *ars, bry, hep, ign, ipec, lyc, nux, phos, puls, sep, sil, sul*

  but cannot vomit *nux*

neck, stiff *caust, cimi, phyt, rhus t*

nervous *acon, arg n, caust, chin, cimi, gels, ign, lach, nux, phos, puls, sil, sul*

nervous system affected *arg n, gels, lach, nux, phos, sil*

neuralgia *see* pain, neuralgic

nightmares *see* dreams, distressing

nosebleeds *arn, chin, ipec, phos*

obsessional *ars, nux, puls, sil*

obstinate *arn, calc, sil*

orderly *ars, kali, nat m, nux*

osteoporosis *calc c, calc fl, calc phos, sil, symph,* 103

ovarian pain *apis, bell, lach, lyc, merc*

overwork *arg n, arn, nux, sep, sil*

pain, bearing down, labour-like *bell, cham, gels, nat m, nux, sep*

  burning *acon, apis, ars, bell, caust, merc, phos,* better for heat *ars*

  cramping *bell, calc, cham, ign, lyc, nux, sul*

  fleeting *bell, ign, phyt, puls*

  intense *bell, cham, cimi*

  neuralgic, shooting *acon, ars, bell, bry, caust, cham, chin, cimi, hep, hyp, ign, lyc, merc, nux, rhus, stap, sul*

  sensitive to *cham, ign, sil, stap*

  spasmodic *bell, ign, nux*

  splinter-like *hep*

  stinging, sudden *apis, ars, merc, sil*

palpitations *acon, arg n, lach, nux, phos, puls,* 106

paralysis *arg n, ars, caust, gels, kali, nux, rhus*

peevish, spiteful *cham, ipec, kali, lach, lyc, nat m, nux, stap, sul*

periods, absent *acon, calc, ign, kali, lach, nat m, puls,* 63

  aggravated before *apis, ars, calc, caust, cham, cimi, kali, lach, lyc, nat m, nux, puls, sep, sul*

  delayed at puberty *calc, kali, nat m, puls, sil,* 61, 63

  irregular *cimi, ign, ipec, nat m, nux, puls, sep*

  painful (dysmenorrhoea) *bell, caul, cham, cimi, col, ign, ipec, kali, lach, lyc, nux, phyt, puls, sep,* 62, 66–67

  scanty *nat m, puls, sul*

perspiration *see* sweat

phlebitis *ars, arn, ham,* 108

piles *bell, calc, caust, ham, kali, lach, nux, puls, sep, sul,* 78

PMS 63–66 *see* periods, aggravated before

pneumonia *kali, lyc*

potencies 41, 42, 43

pregnancy 75–6

pressure aggravates *acon, apis, arg n, ars, bell, calc, hep, kali, lach, lyc, nux, phos, sil*

phos, puls, sul

heat aggravates *apis, arg n, arn, bell, bry, gels, ipec, kali, lach, lyc, nat m, merc, sul*

warm damp, humid aggravates *gels, lach, nat m, puls, rhus*

  ameliorates *caust, cham, hep, sil*

warm dry ameliorates *nux, sil*

warm-blooded *apis, arg n, bell, sul*

warm stuffy aggravates *acon, apis, arg n, bry, lyc, puls*

thirst *see* food

throat, choking sensation *bell, caus, ign, lach*

  hoarseness *bell, caus, phos*

  sensation of lump in *ign, lach, puls*

  sensitive *lach, phos*

  sore *acon, apis, bell, caust, hep, lach, merc, nux, phos, phyt, puls, rhus, sul*

thrush *borax, merc, nat m, puls, sep,* 69

thundery weather aggravates *phos, phyt*

tics *arg n, ars, ign, nux*

tight bandaging, clothing aggravates *lach, lyc*

  ameliorates *bry, nat m*

timid *ars, caust, chin, gels, kali, lyc, puls, sil*

tinnitus *see* Ménières disease

tongue, shows marks of teeth *merc*

  thick yellow coating *merc*

tonsillitis *bell, calc, hep, lach, merc, phyt, stap*

toothache *cham, ipec, stap*

touch aggravates *acon, apis, arn, bell, bry, chin, hep, lach, sep, stap*

  ameliorates *phos*

touchy, offended, criticized, feels *ars, bry, calc, cham, chin, hep, ign, lach, lyc, nux, puls, sil, stap, sul*

travel, seasickness *ars, ipec*

trembling *arg n, caust, gels, merc, stap*

twitching *ign, nux*

ulceration *arg n, merc, nux*

urethritis *bell, canth, merc, phos, sul*

urination, desire for *bry, canth, caus, merc, nux, pul, stap, sul*

  frequent *caust, gels, lyc, merc, nux, stap, sul*

  involuntary *caust, nat m, phos, puls, rhus*

  painful *acon, canth, cham, merc, nux, pul, stap, sul*

urticaria *apis, sul, urt*

vaginal dryness *bry, cal, lyc, nat m, sep, stap,* 102

vaginitis *ars, calc, puls*

varicose ulcers *cal cream, lach*

varicose veins *arn, ars, bell, calc, carb v, ham, lach, lyc, nux, puls, sep, stap, sul,* 78, 109

vertigo *arn, bell, bry, caust, chin, con, phos,* 109

voice, loss of *arg n, caust, phos*

vomiting, frequent *ars, nux, puls*

weakness, prostration *arg n, arn, ars, carb v, caust, gels, kali, lyc, phos, phyt, sep, sil*

weather *see* temperature

weight, tendency to overweight *calc, kali, puls*

  tendency to underweight *lyc, phos, sil*

wet, getting aggravates *bell* (head), *puls* (feet), *sep*

whitlows *hep, sil*

whooping cough *arn, ipec*

wind aggravates *calc, ham, hep, nux, phos*

wounds, puncture *hyp, led, stap,* 95

yawning *ign, kali*